# Dr. Jordan Metzl's
# WORKOUT
# PRESCRIPTION

## Also by Dr. Jordan Metzl:

*The Young Athlete*

*The Athlete's Book of Home Remedies*

*The Exercise Cure*

*Dr. Jordan Metzl's Running Strong*

# Dr. Jordan Metzl's
# WORKOUT PRESCRIPTION

---

## 10, 20 & 30-MINUTE
## HIGH-INTENSITY
## INTERVAL TRAINING
## WORKOUTS
### for Every Fitness Level

---

# JORDAN D. METZL, MD
### with Mike Zimmerman

RODALE.

## RODALE
# *wellness*

*Live happy. Be healthy. Get inspired.*

Sign up today to get exclusive access to our authors, exclusive bonuses,
and the most authoritative, useful, and cutting-edge information on health,
wellness, fitness, and living your life to the fullest.

**Visit us online at RodaleWellness.com**
**Join us at RodaleWellness.com/Join**

Rodale books may be purchased for business or promotional use or for special sales. For information, please write to:
Special Markets Department, Rodale Inc., 733 Third Avenue, New York, NY 10017.

Printed in the United States of America

Rodale Inc. makes every effort to use acid-free ⊗, recycled paper ♻.

Photo on page v: Dr. Jordan Metzl; page viii bottom: Sara Cedar Miller/Central Park Conservancy;
all other photos: Matt Rainey/Rodale Images
Exercise illustrations: Kagan McLeod
Medical illustrations: Amanda Williams
Book design by Christina Gaugler

Library of Congress Cataloging-in-Publication Data is on file with the publisher
ISBN 978–1–62336–586–8 paperback

Distributed to the trade by Macmillan
2  4  6  8  10  9  7  5  3  1   paperback

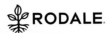

We inspire health, healing, happiness, and love in the world.
Starting with you.

*Five years ago, I started a community-based fitness class called Ironstrength.*

*What started out with 20 people in the basement of a gym has grown into a*

*movement of many thousands of people who join our free, physician-led fitness*

*classes every year. This book is dedicated to the amazing people who have worked*

*out with me, sharing their sweat, smiles, and joy with our Ironstrength community.*

*Together we have built a fitness family.*

*You have made me a better doctor and a better fitness instructor and have helped*

*create a community that continues to nourish everyone who participates.*

*Thanks to you, I've been able to join the worlds of fitness and medicine together*

*to promote health, wellness, and prevention. I dedicate this book to each of you,*

*my friends and workout partners.*

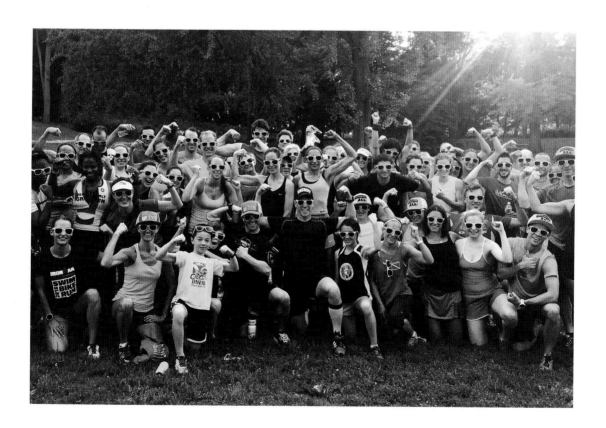

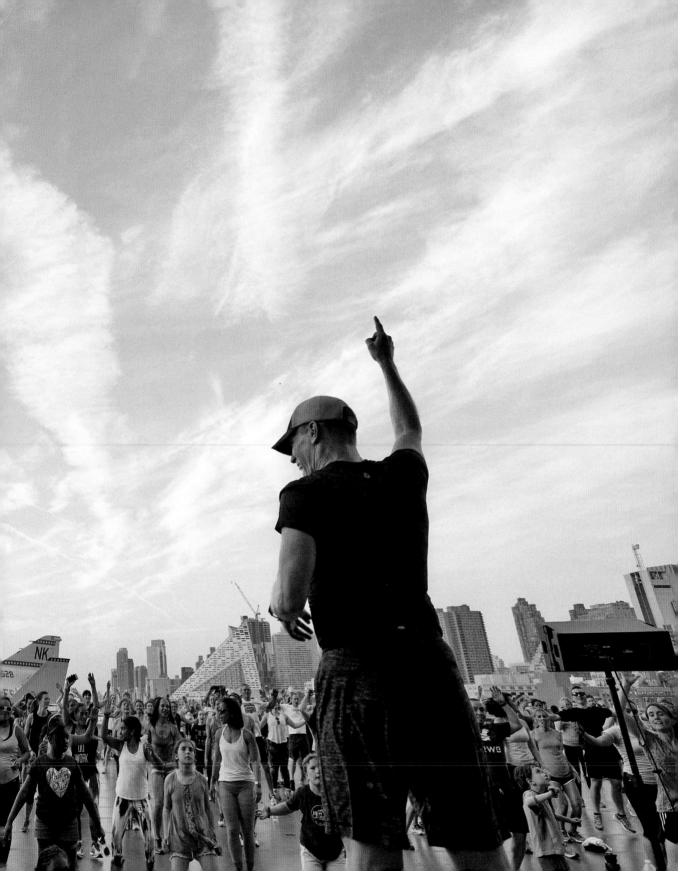

# CONTENTS

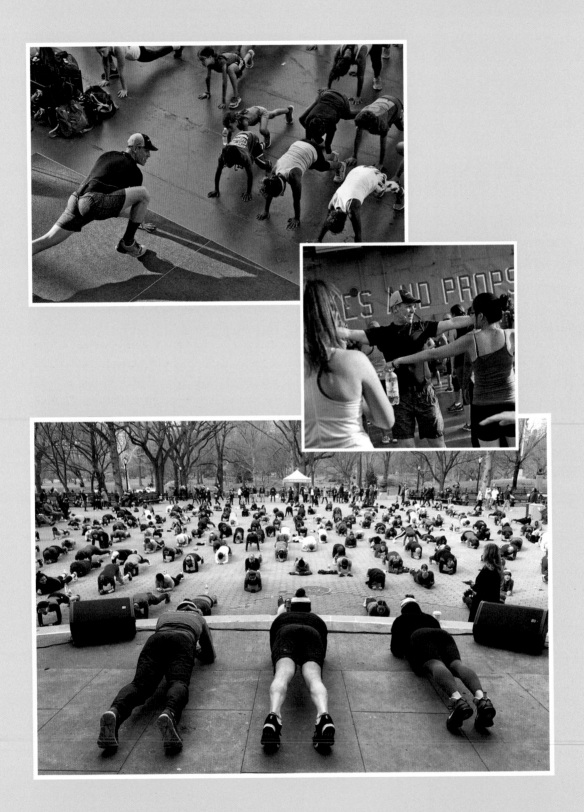

# INTRODUCTION

# We've Come a Long Way!

When I graduated from medical school more than 20 years ago, I hoped I'd be able to help improve the lives of my patients by practicing medicine in an office or hospital, like many doctors do. That sounded gratifying to me, since I come from a family of doctors and knew since I was 5 years old that I'd follow in the family business.

When the time came to choose a specialty, I picked sports medicine because I am an athlete myself and understand that movement is joy—at its core, true joy—and I wanted to keep people moving the way they were meant to. If you had asked me back then if that would be enough, I might have said yes (then again, maybe not—I was fired up back then and still am!). But I've learned through the years that as important as my work in my regular practice is, my role as doctor has evolved in many positive ways that I never anticipated when I first started my journey.

For a long time, I considered my athletic endeavors—like training for triathlons—and my medical career to be separate activities. You could make an appointment to see me at the office for your achy hip or knee, but if you wanted to see me any other time, you'd have to flag me down while I was out running or cycling. Exercise was my private island.

That's pretty much how most people live their lives: *I work during the day; I do my other thing on nights and weekends.*

But then things began to change.

I published *The Athlete's Book of Home Remedies*, which was designed to keep active people moving by offering information on diagnosing, treating, and preventing common sports injuries. It was successful and reached more people in 1 month than I could ever have seen in my entire career of office practice. That's powerful.

Two years later, I published *The Exercise Cure: A Doctor's All-Natural, No-Pill Prescription for Better Health & Longer Life.* As you can see from the title, the book was designed to help people prevent or improve a vast number of health problems—from annoying issues like fatigue all the way up to the most serious conditions, like heart disease and certain cancers—using exercise. This second book really started narrowing the gap between my worlds of exercise and medicine. *The Exercise Cure* was even more successful than *The Athlete's Book of Home Remedies* and once again extended my reach to many thousands of people beyond the borders of New York City, where I work as a sports medicine physician at Hospital for Special

Surgery, and even beyond the borders of the United States.

That led to a dream project of mine, a book with *Runner's World* titled *Dr. Jordan Metzl's Running Strong,* and my first workout DVD, called *The Ironstrength Workout for Runners.* These two projects collected all the helpful things I'd learned not just as a doctor but also as a dedicated (and perhaps a little fanatical!) runner. At last, all the things I wanted to tell runners—about health, injury, and prevention—were collected in one place. I've also done a series of instructional videos for *Runner's World* magazine (runnersworld .com), and I've worked to get content across multiple platforms to reach an ever-broadening audience. The goal, as always, is to keep athletes moving through education and smarter training.

As I look back at my path, I see that my loves of exercise and medicine had always been merging—I just didn't fully realize it at the time. Over the years, I've learned more and more about my field, how our bodies work, and how my own body responds to new and different forms of exercise. As far as endurance training—all that running, biking, and swimming—I figured I had that down. When I discovered HIIT (high-intensity interval training), however, it was like a whole new world of health, fitness, and performance opened up. HIIT training made everything better—not just my race times but also how I felt day to day: stronger, healthier, more energetic (and that's saying something) and with fewer aches and pains, especially in my joints. Why did I feel so good? The muscle I built helped support my joints and connective tissue and also let me work longer and at a higher level.

I was so won over by that style of training that I began teaching free classes on the weekends to help my patients and area athletes benefit from the same strength gains that had helped me succeed. I recognized that it was much more fun to do this kind of training with a crowd, so why not create one? I doubt many MDs moonlight as group fitness instructors, but this was really one of the most apparent ways that exercise and medical practice began to merge for me. Once again, I saw a way to help more and more people maximize their movement and raise their quality of life. Over time, medicine for me became as much about preventing disease and injury as it was about fixing achy knees, shoulders, and backs.

Then a funny thing happened. As time went by, the free classes (called Ironstrength Community Fitness Classes) got bigger. Twenty people became 30, and so on. Soon I would regularly see a hundred or more people in my outdoor Central Park classes. And it doesn't get any better than August 2015, when I ran an Ironstrength class for more than *a thousand people* on the deck of the aircraft carrier USS *Intrepid* under the Manhattan skyline on the Hudson River. I've run several of these massive *Intrepid* classes since, and they've become semiregular events covered by national news outlets.

Throughout this evolution, technology has helped connect an ever-growing network of like-minded fitness enthusiasts via e-mail newsletters and social media. People were talkin'. Fast-forward to today: Together we've built a freestanding Ironstrength fitness community of thousands that helps athletes of all ages and levels, from 10-year-old kids to

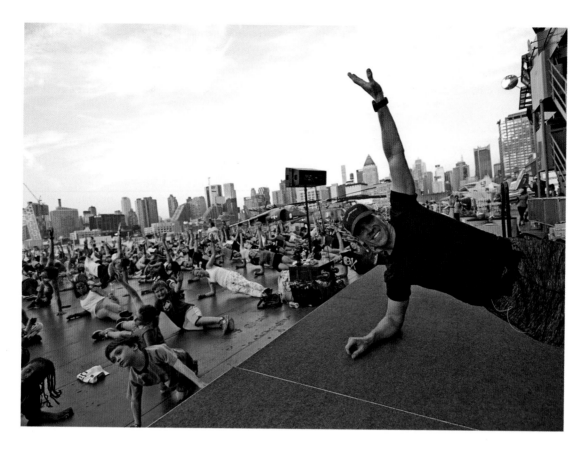

81-year-old grandmothers, build fitness and strength in unison. The most amazing thing about this group is how its members have grown to support and care for each other. When we meet in the middle of New York City, we create a flash mob of sweat, smiles, and support.

Our Ironstrength community workouts have led to greater opportunities to reach a broader audience as I've also been invited by national media outlets like the *Today* show to help viewers across the country move more, get stronger, and feel better. The concept of a physician-led fitness program is catching on, and I hope to spread this concept around the country.

On a one-on-one basis in my medical practice, the exercise-medicine merger is complete. Exercise is a vital part of how I practice. I still do the usual "doctoring" during an appointment—analyze complaint, diagnose problem, prescribe remedy—but exercise is a regular part of the prescription process. And that's for everyone I see at all ages and fitness levels. We've even started a curriculum to teach medical students how to best prescribe exercise to their patients.

Why do I do this? Science validates the medical benefits of exercise—you'll read more about that shortly—but anecdotally, I see terrific results in my patients. That's the bottom line. Increasing activity affects all areas of their lives, from how they age to what sports they participate in and, indeed, what they're physically capable of overall. I also see the results in myself. Strength training helped my endurance training. It really is that simple. If you make an appointment to see me in the office, no matter what your malady, exercise will almost always be part of the conversation. It's the safest and most effective drug known to humankind, a magic pill that I love to prescribe.

Going back to that day I graduated from medical school, did I foresee a time when I could be helping millions of people instead of the thousands I'd see in my office over my career? No. As motivated as I was, that wet-behind-the-ears MD could not have foreseen what's possible.

This all brings us to the book you're now holding in your hands, *Dr. Jordan Metzl's Workout Prescription*. This book has a personal history. When my last book was published, a reader in New York wrote me a note: "Dr. Metzl, I love your information and I'd love to do a marathon someday, but I have to be realistic. I have three kids, a job, and a commute. I have 20 to 30 minutes per day to exercise. How about something for me?" Around the same time, I began researching the science of HIIT and realized that if done properly, 20 to 30 minutes of high-intensity exercise can be as valuable as 60 minutes of less-intense exercise. The concept here is simple: If you're time crunched, I want you to get the most out of your fitness routine. This book is designed for the readers around the world who have precious little time, and sometimes not even a gym, and need to maximize their dose of the medicine of exercise.

*Dr. Jordan Metzl's Workout Prescription* applies everything I've learned as a sports medicine doctor, an athlete, and a fitness instructor to help you get regular, beneficial exercise into your life as quickly and easily as possible. Most people have 30 minutes. But even if you have just 10, I've got you covered and you'll still see benefits. Just move! Most of the workouts require little to no equipment. All you have to do is turn the page.

Standing here today, I feel so lucky to be in a position to help people understand the healthiest and most effective ways to move. I'm more motivated than ever to get the message out there—that movement is joy, that exercise is medicine (for the body and the soul), and that the cheapest, easiest, and most certain way to feel better and live longer is simply to break a sweat. No matter what your age, I hope you find these workouts beneficial as you strive to become the healthiest version of yourself.

If you're holding this book, you're now part of our community. Welcome aboard! Every time you huff and puff, remember that somewhere around the world, someone else is doing the same thing. You're now on my team! Ready to roll? Let's get started!

—*Jordan D. Metzl, MD*
*Hospital for Special Surgery*
*New York City*

# PART ONE

# Are You Missing the Big (Fitness) Picture?

**M**any people, from those just getting off the couch to others who have done a specific kind of workout for years, have preconceived notions about exercise. They also have their own reasons for exercising (or not exercising). In my role as a physician, I talk to a lot of people about this—asking them why they exercise and what they think is the best way—and I hear the same variety of answers: They enjoy one particular exercise. Or they want to lose weight. Or they want to complete (insert athletic event here). Or they want to achieve the perfect (insert body part here). On the surface, good answers, right? Anything that motivates a person to move is a good thing. But if I can make one suggestion to these people, it's this: Your reason isn't big enough. For sure, I want you to love exercise or lose weight or have a great butt. But what if you could have all those things and even more? That's what I mean about thinking big. And that's why this first section of the book will show you three steps to your newer, bigger, better workout plan.

## CHAPTER ONE

# STEP 1: IT'S NOT ABOUT TIME
## (Though 30 Minutes Is a Sweet Spot!)

Time is a funny thing. It flies. It drags. And yet time is the same every time. Sixty seconds in every minute, 60 minutes in every hour, and so on. That means that after 30 minutes, you've burned 1,800 seconds, whether you were standing in line to get a driver's license photo or watching your favorite TV comedy. The only difference is how each of those 1,800 seconds felt as it ticked away.

In other words, how you fill the time ultimately determines what you get out of it.

If you happen to be on the phone with a friend you haven't spoken with in a year, you won't even realize there's a wait for that driver's license photo. Meanwhile, if that episode of your favorite show is a rerun, your mind may wander and time will pass more slowly.

Time is like that for just about every activity, but nothing gives people more fits than time partnered with exercise. Consider:

■ What's the most common thing you hear about exercise? "I don't have time."

■ Packing a bag, driving to the gym, changing, working out, cooling down, showering (hopefully!), changing again, and returning to your day—all represent little pockets of time. They add up.

■ What about those seconds ticking away during a workout? Well, let's just say that some seconds tick faster than others. (I can vouch for that: Mile 2 of a marathon ticks away a lot faster than, say, Mile 22.)

■ And then there's the biggest issue of all, the problem this book was designed to solve: *How much time do you really need to exercise effectively?*

The answer? Well, I'm not sure a definitive answer exists. The science is pretty clear in that the health benefits level off at around 150 minutes per week of moderate activity, which equates to 30 minutes of brisk walking 5 days a week. That's a solid recommendation, and it makes 30 minutes one kind of sweet spot. But is it definitive? Nope. Someone who wants to run a marathon needs more exercise than someone who just wants to enjoy a Spinning class with friends. Still, if you want to feel better, improve your health,

# Know Before You Go (This Is Important!)

I recommend that anyone who wants to ramp up his or her exercise activity see a doctor for a full physical beforehand. This is especially true for anyone who has been inactive for a while or is over age 40 (or both). Let the doc know what you have planned and that you want to know that the machine is in good working order before you start. This isn't a disclaimer—this is smart medical advice for several reasons.

■ Your doctor can give you a thorough going-over, including examining your medical history. This is especially crucial if you've had past physical issues like chest pain, dizziness, or even joint pain.

■ Your doctor can help guide your fitness plan. She's probably not a trainer, but she can give you advice on how hard you should go based on your physical condition. And listen to her. One thing about gung-ho humans: Their eyes are bigger than their stomachs (and muscles and cardiovascular fitness level).

■ You'll establish baseline numbers for your blood pressure, cholesterol, and all those other wonderful markers you should have memorized but probably don't. Improving your fitness generally improves your health stats. Don't you want to know how well you're doing? That's part of the payoff!

build strength, and live a more active lifestyle, you need very little time to exercise. In fact, it comes down to the title of this chapter: To get real benefits from exercise, it's not about time. It's about what you put into the time you have—the types of exercises and the intensity with which you perform them. Once you master that concept, the clock becomes a very good friend indeed.

## INTENSITY, EFFICIENCY, TOTALITY

This book promises 30-minute workouts—and you'll find a bunch of them in here—but the fact is, you can do the 10- and 20-minute versions and still enjoy health benefits, build muscle, and increase your overall fitness. How? Again, it's about intensity and volume—how hard you work and how much work you do in a given time period.

I'm a big endurance sports guy. I run marathons and do Ironman triathlons. Those are timed events, which means that the better I perform in a race, the shorter that race is for me. (Now there's some incentive to swim, run, and pedal faster—it'll all be over sooner.) But if you have a set time for a workout, it's kind of like an empty box on moving day. You could toss a bunch of stuff into it and put it on the truck, but then you'd probably need more empty boxes to get the end result you want, which is all your stuff on the truck.

But what if you learned how to pack the box more efficiently? To use all the space in the box? And do it in half the time? You'd get all your stuff on the truck in one shot and boom, you'd be done.

That's what this book will help you do. How? By focusing on intensity, efficiency, and totality.

■ **Intensity.** The workouts in this book (whether 10 minutes, 20 minutes, or 30 minutes) consist of high-intensity interval training, or HIIT. You may have heard of HIIT. We'll discuss it in more detail shortly, but the bottom line is that HIIT workouts deliver incredible performance results—you'll be better, stronger, and faster, for sure—but also serious, research-backed health benefits. The ever-expanding science of HIIT shows that you can achieve better physical, mental, and physiological results if you're able to master this type of workout. (I think it's worth it!)

■ **Efficiency.** Most of the exercises in the 30-minute workouts are designed to work multiple muscles across a series of compound movements. A single-movement exercise like a biceps curl is just fine for your biceps, but not very efficient for the rest of your body. If you can engage dozens of muscles in 5 seconds versus just a few muscles, which strategy gets more done? Using the moving box analogy, these exercises pack more activity and muscle engagement into a smaller space (or time, as it were).

■ **Totality.** I'm all about total-body fitness. Yes, I offer some targeted workouts for your core, lower body, and upper body later in the book, but the overall mission is building your entire body in a balanced way to help

## Why I Believe Exercising 7 Days a Week Is an Awesome Idea

Exercising 7 days a week sounds extreme, but it really isn't. Some people out there would immediately say, "No way—your body needs time to recover. Why would a doctor recommend something so crazy?"

It's pretty simple: I believe the human body is designed for everyday use. We're mobile creatures. Sofas are a relatively new invention. Just look back a hundred years, five hundred, a thousand, and more. Our ancestors, from the caves to the farm fields, got their butts out the door early and sweated all day, every day. The difference is they did it because they had to, without any real knowledge of how to take care of themselves and with very little medical care. Well, we can do it because we want to, it's good for us, and we know so much more today (and if you do injure yourself, you probably won't die like in the old days).

The key to daily exercise? Avoiding overuse. How do you do this?

Change it up. Do something different from your normal workouts, and go easier than you normally do. Bring friends. Smile a lot. I call this kind of movement dynamic rest and talk about it in more detail later in the book—with suggestions!

I look at daily exercise as a healthy addiction. We have such an obesity problem and so many obesity-related health issues that are treated after they happen, as opposed to trying to prevent them in the first place. Hypertension and diabetes are preventable and potentially reversible with daily exercise. Exercise is medicine, preventive medicine, and I believe it should be a daily ritual just like brushing your teeth.

My point is, a body that is used sensibly every day grows accustomed to being used and won't be as prone to injury.

it perform better and prevent injury. Oh, and your day-to-day life will be easier—from climbing stairs to hauling laundry. Total-body fitness leads to total-life payoffs.

## SCORE YOUR FIRST BIG HIIT (OR, HOW MANY PLAYS ON THE TERM *HIIT* CAN WE FIT INTO ONE BOOK?)

Interval training isn't new. Runners have a classic German term for it—*fartlek*—which has inspired jokes among high school cross-country teammates for decades. People who use intervals in any kind of training know how well they work.

So what is HIIT? It's simple: Instead of exercising at one pace for an extended period of time—think jogging 3 miles on a Saturday morning—you work at a higher intensity for short intervals of time (thus the name) with rest periods figured in. So a runner, for example, would run at a much faster pace for, say, 30 seconds, then dial it back for a minute, and then ramp back up for 30 seconds more, etc. That's a very basic example; there are limitless ways you can break up intervals and rest periods, and you can apply the concept to any activity (even bowling, though that would be . . . strange).

Steady-state cardio exercises like running are good for you—fantastic, even—and do challenge your body. However, over long periods, they ultimately train your physique to be more efficient. Think how elite distance runners have more compact frames—their bodies have been trained to use energy more efficiently; therefore, their muscles have adapted to be smaller to consume fewer resources for the effort exerted.

Now consider the sprinter: bigger muscles, more explosive fast-twitch fibers, built not for long-haul efficiency but for short-burst intensity. Sprinters by default use interval training because they need that all-out, leave-nothing-in-the-tank effort to get to the finish line first.

That's HIIT in a nutshell. But what does it do for you? And how does it do it?

Working at the high-intensity level raises your heart rate and increases your body's oxygen consumption. This can lead to burning more calories and fat. In fact, your body continues consuming oxygen after the workout is over, sometimes for hours. This is known as excess post-exercise oxygen consumption, or EPOC. I use this concept all the time in my office. I talk to my patients about turning on their "metabolic furnace" for the day by using intensity first thing in the morning. Exactly how many more calories are burned? It's difficult to calculate—every person's body is different—but it can be as high as 25 to 30 percent more, compared with steady-state workouts, according to the American College of Sports Medicine.

So: shorter workouts, higher oxygen and calorie burn, better total-body fitness. Not a bad collection of benefits. But like a bad infomercial—wait! There's more!

HIIT has been around long enough that researchers have had time to study its various effects on the body, and I expect more research to pile up as the years go by, since HIIT is a rich subject. Aside from considering all the information I've just given you, have a look at some of the scientifically tested benefits of adding HIIT strength sessions to your regular exercise regimen (or, if you're fresh off the couch and just starting, why HIIT should be part of whatever you're planning to try, be it a simple walking program or something more ambitious). I think you'll be happy you did.

### HIIT–specifically, with strength training–helps deliver a bigger burn.

I touched on this just now, but we haven't talked about the benefits of strength training (as opposed to steady-state cardio like running or cycling). A small study in the journal *Medicine and Science in Sports and Exercise*[1] monitored the oxygen consumption (known as $VO_2$ max, a measurement based on body weight and lung capacity) of 15 men as they performed interval-style weight training for 27 minutes, and then, 5 days later, ran steady-state on treadmills to achieve identical $VO_2$ levels for 27 minutes. In other words, they did weight training and treadmill running at the same effort level for the same amount of time. The result? Total oxygen consumption was higher for 30 minutes after the weight-training workout.

Another study—this time of seven women ages 22 to 35, in the *International Journal of Sport Nutrition and Exercise Metabolism*,[2]—showed elevated metabolic rate for 3 hours after an intense resistance workout, compared with pre-exercise levels. To boot, resting fat oxidation was elevated 2 days after the workout.

That's exciting stuff. HIIT has long been thought to help boost metabolism and "afterburn." Still, some data have shown that the fitter you are, the lower your EPOC. A study of 10 men in the journal *BMC Research Notes* in 2012[3] showed just that—though this study looked at cardio, not strength training.

These are small studies and just examples of what kind of research has been going on in the world of HIIT, but they give a glimpse of the overall potential benefits. In conclusion, the harder you work, the more physiologically efficient you'll become, achieving better results in less time.

## What about Cardio?

I compare HIIT to steady-state cardio a lot in this chapter. That doesn't mean I'm anti-cardio. I run, bike, and swim more than most folks as I train for Ironman triathlons. I love those activities and wouldn't give them up for anything. They bring unbelievable mental and physical rewards. But as much as I want to do them, I want to have total-body fitness. I want the strength and flexibility that HIIT gives me. And my HIIT workouts have improved my steady-state performance. There's no downside.

But here's another reason I love HIIT for strength: You work your muscles, but you also work at an intensity high enough to give you a first-rate cardio challenge while simultaneously building strength. My patients often ask, "Is this a strength day or a cardio day?" The truth is that when you do HIIT, it's just a day. You're building both strength and cardiopulmonary fitness at the same time. You can do nothing but these workouts a few times a week and get yourself stronger and in great cardiovascular shape. Now that's a comprehensive workout.

# Can a 10-Minute Workout Really Deliver Health and Fitness Benefits?

Yes, it can. Research has begun to consistently bear this out: A recent study in the journal *PLOS ONE*[4] had otherwise-healthy obese participants perform 3 minutes of intense intermittent exercise within a 30-minute weekly training time commitment for 6 weeks (three sessions of 10 minutes that included 1 minute of intervals per week). The results: improved oxygen consumption, lower blood pressure, and increased insulin sensitivity.

And that was just from adding *1 minute* of intense exercise in a 10-minute training window three times a week.

Another *PLOS ONE* study[5] analyzed a 12-week interval program with 53 sedentary men. They improved their cardiometabolic health indices as much as they would have by doing traditional endurance exercise, but with a fivefold lower time commitment.

Now, my mentioning two small studies is one thing. But I believe that if you have a normally low or moderate activity level and you start doing 10-minute HIIT strength workouts three times a week, you'll know how beneficial they are just by how you feel. And if you make a commitment to measure body markers like blood pressure, resting heart rate, and blood sugar before you begin (ask your doctor), and then again after 6 weeks, you'll see a measurable difference.

## HIIT might help control your blood sugar and appetite.

For overweight and obese people, prediabetes and full-blown type 2 diabetes are realities. Many doctors call it an epidemic and the biggest and most expensive health issue of our time. That's no exaggeration. If your body isn't processing glucose—the sugar in your bloodstream—correctly, the sweet stuff can damage your tissues. That's why people with diabetes have problems with nerve pain, blurred vision, vascular damage, and potentially worse outcomes like heart disease. It's a painful and dangerous condition to live with if it's not controlled.

Well, guess what? Exercise, especially HIIT, may help control and improve blood glucose readings and insulin sensitivity and maybe even decrease your appetite.

A 2015 study in the journal *PLOS ONE*[6] showed that after undergoing an 8-week interval exercise program, working out three times per week, participants with type 2 diabetes showed significantly lower blood glucose and increased insulin sensitivity, as well as abdominal fat loss. Great news all around. Meanwhile, a 2013 review of six studies in the journal *Diabetes Metabolic Syndrome and Obesity*[7] found that even brief high-intensity interval training—sometimes less than 2 minutes per exercise session—led to improved blood glucose levels for 1 to 3 days after the workout in both people with type 2 diabetes and those who don't have the condition.

And here's something you might never have heard of before: Nesfatin is a chemical (a neuropeptide, to be specific) produced in your brain that helps regulate appetite. The more you have, the less hungry you feel. And a 2015 study in the *Journal of Hormone and Molecular Biology Clinical Investigation*[8] found that after a three-session-per-week training program lasting 6 weeks, nesfatin-1 levels increased in participants who did HIIT but not in people who did moderate-intensity continuous exercise.

Pretty cool, right?

If you're overweight and sedentary and coming to this book for help, this section right here is the best argument for adding a HIIT component to your life. It may seem too challenging or intimidating or even unattainable, but it isn't. All you have to do is get up and start. And keep reading! There's even more good news ahead.

## Chances are, you'll like HIIT better than other workouts.

Sound far-fetched? Not really. How much a person enjoys a workout will determine how often she does it (which shows you how much I truly enjoy running, cycling, swimming, and interval strength training—the kid can't get enough!). But will you really dig HIIT for

## And Now a Word about Women and Muscles

I can only speak from my own experience, and there's no way to verify it, but I believe that the positive message about women and strength training has finally turned the corner. I now know so many women who are regular strength trainers that it no longer seems novel or like some kind of breakthrough. For years, all I'd hear (and read) was that women don't want to build muscle. The reasons were varied, but most sounded something like "Women don't want to train like men" or "Women don't want to bulk up." Well, those two myths have been severely debunked. The only reason resistance workouts meant "training like men" was because men were the ones training that way. Now that women have caught on, it's just plain old training. As for bulking up, well, the only way that happens is if you want to train like a football lineman or a bodybuilder. And those very different training methods require specific regimens (including diet) to get results. Furthermore, men have much higher levels of testosterone, which leads to greater muscle hypertrophy and growth, compared with women. Physiologically, men build more muscle bulk than women. So unless you set out with one of those goals in mind, it just ain't gonna happen. Regular strength training, however, will deliver all the benefits you'll read about in this book. And last time I checked, women benefit from well-trained muscles just as much as any man does. A 2015 study in the journal *Applied Physiology, Nutrition, and Metabolism*[9] compared HIIT strength training with HIIT rowing to see how female bodies responded to both. Twenty-eight women participated for 6 weeks. Cardio fitness improvements were similar in both styles of exercise. However, the strength trainers saw "significant" increases in squat, press, and deadlift performance, as well as in the broad jump, while the rowers saw no increases.

It's intuitive: Strength training makes you stronger. But many women resisted that message for years. From what I see, the pendulum has swung the other way, and that's a great thing for health; positive body image; and bone, muscle, tendon, and ligament strength.

# Have You Heard about Tabata?

Tabata is a particularly intense form of interval training developed in Japan that's not for the faint of heart. It's pretty simple: Whatever your activity, go at it hard for 20 seconds, rest for 10, and repeat for 8 sets without stopping. That's 4 minutes. I promise you, if you go full bore on each sprint, this will be one of the most difficult workouts you'll ever do. Try it only after your body is warmed up and prepared for maximum effort, maybe after one of your regular workouts. *Important:* Whatever activity you do for Tabata training (and this is true of any exercise), never sacrifice form. The point is to work out safely and effectively. The second your form breaks down, you increase your chance of injury, so back off immediately. Build slowly. Be smart.

strength more than any other workouts you do? It's possible. A 2014 study in *PLOS ONE*[10] compared HIIT-style workouts with "continuous moderate" and "continuous vigorous" intensity exercise. Researchers administered those types of workouts randomly among 44 people, stretched out over four different sessions. The result: More than half of the people preferred HIIT over the other types of exercise.

Why? It might have something to do with this next item.

### HIIT may feel easier than other workouts.

That's not a bad selling point, right? Well, research points in that direction. The American College of Sports Medicine's journal, *Medicine and Science in Sports and Exercise*, published a 2015 study[11] comparing "rate of perceived exertion," or RPE, between continuous exercise and interval training. Twenty sedentary people (11 men, 9 women) took part, and the researchers arrived at two interesting results: First, the folks doing intervals had a lower RPE, compared with the continuous exercise group—in short, intervals felt easier, even though the actual intensity was identical between the two groups and the interval trials lasted longer. Second, among the interval group, participants felt that shorter, more frequent intervals were easier, compared with longer, less-frequent ones. In other words, the shorter the interval, the easier the session felt, *even when intensity was the same across all workouts.*

This is huge. It's a small study, but the researchers worked with folks who don't normally exercise—which is the majority of society—and HIIT workouts felt easiest and so may be more appealing than other types of exercise. My take? If you haven't tried a HIIT workout, you may be missing out on a type of exercise that will not just do you a world of good but that you also could fall in love with (or at least like enough to do more!).

### HIIT could make you better at other workouts.

I've mentioned this before. This is one of my favorite benefits, and it's one of the reasons I've embraced HIIT strength workouts so wholeheartedly. They just make you better at everything else. Scandinavian researchers have taken a good look at this phenomenon over the years, publishing a number of studies showing the effects of HIIT and strength training on steady-state exercises like running and cycling. A 2015 study in the *Scandinavian Journal of Medicine and Science in Sports*[12] found that adding HIIT training (though not strength training) to the regimens of 132 recreational runners improved their 5K times, as well as lowered the blood pressure of hypertensive subjects. The control group, not surprisingly, saw no changes.

Another study from the KIHU Research Institute for Olympic Sports in Finland[13] looked at the effects of strength training on recreational runners. Twenty-seven men completed an 8-week program of three types of training (heavy resistance, explosive resistance, and muscle endurance). All three groups improved their treadmill-running endurance. The heavy and explosive training modes gave the biggest muscle-building benefits, while the heavy mode gave the most high-intensity-running benefit.

And finally, another study from the *Scandinavian Journal of Medicine and Science in Sports*[14] found that adding strength training to the normal endurance training of 14 elite cyclists improved both short-term (5-minute) and long-term (45-minute) time-trial endurance, as well as muscle fiber size and strength.

## A FEW MORE THINGS BEFORE YOU HIIT IT

When you're approaching a HIIT workout—especially for the first time—you're basically trying to answer four questions.

1. **How long should I work?** It depends on your fitness level. Some folks can work longer than others. One way to find out: Start with a 10-minute HIIT session based on the approach in Part Four and see how you feel. Starting out, most people err on the gung-ho side and do too much, too soon. That's normal, and there's a beautiful, built-in natural cure for this: Your body will tell you everything you need to know.

## How Often Should I HIIT It?

Full disclosure: HIIT workouts, especially the strength-training workouts in this book, are challenging. My 30-minute workouts are adjustable to fit the challenge you need, but if you do them right, your body will need some recovery time. How much? Only you can answer that, based on your fitness level and how you feel. My advice: Start slow. Do one of these workouts per week for 2 or 3 weeks at first. See how you feel a couple of days after each workout. If you feel like your body is ready to go again, add a second workout a week. That's enough for most people to see real improvement in strength and flexibility. Those who want the extra challenge can go three times a week, but I'd cap it at that—*and never do these workouts on consecutive days.* You need to allow your body time to recover and give yourself an opportunity to do other things.

**2. How hard should I work?** This is the *HI* in *HIIT*, so we're looking for high intensity. You can quantify that in different ways. Generally, a high-intensity workout is considered to be 80 percent of your maximum effort sustained for the given interval (fitter people may be able to approach 95 to 100 percent of maximum). You can guesstimate that and do just fine: Carrying on a conversation should be difficult to impossible. Simple, right? However, if you want to be more precise, I recommend using a heart rate monitor. (See "How to Train with a Heart Rate Monitor" below for specifics.)

**3. How long should I rest?** These 30-minute workouts are timed, so a set rest period is literally baked into each minute (you'll get more specific details and instructions in the workout section).

**4. How should I rest?** If you're busting your butt—yet just starting out—you'll want and need the rest, period. In fact, you'll probably need to just stand, hands on hips, and breathe. That's fine—give your body what it wants. However, if you have a higher fitness level, you might want to fill the rest period with some other activity— jogging in place, jumping jacks, or some other exercise you can transition into instantly—that you do anywhere up to 50 percent of maximum capacity. Essentially, you should feel comfortable, still working but allowing your body to rebound for the next interval. Your rest is up to you, and again, I urge you to listen to your body and not err on the side of gung-ho. The goal is not just to finish but to finish with a smile.

## How to Train with a Heart Rate Monitor

Heart rate monitors are exactly what they sound like: small devices that measure your heartbeat while you train. They come in a variety of shapes and sizes, some strapping around your chest and others to your wrist. Using them to train is simple: If you want to train at, say, 85 percent of your maximum heart rate (MHR)—which is in the interval range—just calculate your MHR, multiply by 0.85, and then use the monitor to reach and sustain that rate throughout your interval. It really is that easy.

How do you calculate your MHR? For many years, this has been the standard:

220 - (your age) = your MHR

You may find different, more complex formulas out there, especially those designed for very fit, extremely active people (all the way up to elite athletes), but for an average, semiactive person, this one should work just fine.

Once you program your MHR into your device, you'll receive one of the best benefits of using a monitor: It will let you know when you're at your limit and keep you from overdoing it, which is especially good for beginners.

## YOU'VE HEARD THE DO'S; NOW HERE ARE THE DON'TS

I'm a can-do kind of guy, but I also treat can-do patients who maybe went against some smart advice and hurt themselves. So in a book filled with "can-do's," I want to wrap up this first chapter by recapping some important "please-don'ts."

- **Don't** sacrifice form. If you can't hold exercise form through the movement, your body is telling you to back off. Listen!

- **Don't** do these strength workouts on consecutive days. Let your body recover by doing some other activity or taking a rest day.

- **Don't** ignore your body's injury signals. There's a difference between soreness and pain. Check out the injury section in Part Three for more details.

- **Don't** be intimidated by HIIT or by any workout in this book. (You didn't think all the don'ts would be negative, did you? What a bummer that would be.) I made the workouts adaptable so anyone can try them. So try them!

- **Don't** forget to have fun! Movement is a privilege and a blessing, not something you've been sentenced to. Celebrate it!

## CHAPTER TWO

# STEP 2: IT'S NOT ABOUT WEIGHT LOSS

## (But You Probably Will Lose Weight!)

Exercise is linked to weight loss so often, the pair might as well tie the knot. But would it be a happy marriage? That's a really good question. And the answer you get will depend on whom you ask.

- Some experts will tell you that weight loss is 80 percent diet and 20 percent exercise. They're probably right.

- Other experts will tell you that if you run X distance, you'll burn Y calories, and that could help you lose weight. They're probably right, too.

- Yet another expert will tell you that exercise is great for fitness and health but lousy for weight loss. Probably right again.

Is everyone right? Well, in each case I said "probably." Here's an answer that might be more helpful: In just about any scenario where you change the math on calories—burning more than you take in—you'll lose weight. Of course, how you get to that point can vary greatly.

Do you want to lose weight using my 30-minute workouts? You can. But you might not. It's about the calorie math, not which workout you pick. If you don't lose weight, is that a bad thing? Consider: Let's say you want to lose weight and you do an exercise program faithfully for 3 or 4 weeks. You see some results in the mirror—*Hey, I look a little leaner*—but the scale? Hasn't budged. Maybe this makes you angry. *I did this to lose weight!* Well, maybe you traded some fat for muscle without changing your weight (muscle is denser than fat). And maybe you feel stronger. Maybe your resting heart rate and blood pressure dropped. Maybe your metabolism is revved up. Maybe your body is primed for another 3 or 4 weeks of exercise, and you can do more because you're fitter than you were last month.

If all that happened, tell me: Would you still be angry about not losing weight?

That's the thing about exercise and weight loss: lots of correct answers, even more variables, and all of them tied to the expectations of the person trying to lose the pounds.

My advice: Think bigger. Accept that weight loss is only one potential outcome of regular exercise and that some of the other potential outcomes could be just as good or even better for you than weight loss by itself.

As I often tell my patients, it's much healthier to be mildly to moderately overweight and active than very thin and inactive.

That's what this chapter and the next are all about.

## I'M A DRUG DEALER, AND IT'S TIME FOR YOUR FIX

If dealin' drugs is wrong, I don't wanna be right. For years, I've peddled one type in particular, what I call a miracle drug. Taken regularly, this drug can help prevent, improve, or cure a host of medical problems, from the most annoying to the most frightening.

Too good to be true? Hey, this is your dealer talkin'. This drug is also cheap and plentiful, and it has no side effects. Wait—that's a lie. It has many side effects. It'll make you feel good. It'll improve your strength, flexibility, and mobility. You'll jump higher and move faster. Your sex life might improve. You'll sleep better. You could lose weight. It'll make your life better. It'll make it longer, too.

Man, I'm the biggest pusher of this drug. I want you hooked. I want you using every day. I want you looking for your fix as soon as the sun comes up.

Have I broken bad? Am I cookin' my own brand of meth here in New York City? You bet I am. And its street name is exercise. (You knew where I was going with this, right?) If you want to come see this drug in action, join one of our free community Ironstrength classes next time you're in NYC! (You can register for my free classes at DrJordanMetzl .com.)

Everything I just said is true. I view exercise as a miracle drug, and I want as many people on it as possible. The American College of Sports Medicine uses the phrase "exercise is medicine," and I wholeheartedly agree—so much so that it's become a cornerstone of my medical practice. It's not wishful thinking. Thousands of doctors have spent decades researching exercise and treating millions of people for self-inflicted health problems caused by lack of fitness. The result is undisputed: Exercise is real, honest, all-natural medicine that can help prevent, treat, and resolve a host of medical problems. It's also the easiest, cheapest, and fastest way to a happy life. When formerly sedentary people start moving regularly, miraculous things happen—just as miraculous as those I've seen from any treatment or procedure or drug I've ever prescribed in my 15-plus years in the health care field.

And, like I said, I'm your dealer. I can hook you up. I want you to maximize your dose of the world's most effective medicine.

But first, let me show you what I mean.

## WHAT'S REALLY KILLING YOU

When I say, "Exercise is medicine," one of the most common questions I get is, "What does that mean?"

When the media talk about national health problems, obesity is always at the top of the list. And I agree, it's an epidemic and one of the biggest health crises we face. However, my medical experience has taught me that the common denominator among many health problems, major and minor, is a low fitness level. Now, there are plenty of overweight and obese people out there who have low fitness levels, but then, so do a lot of normal-weight folks. Low fitness isn't limited to the overweight and obese.

That's partly why this book is called *Dr. Jordan Metzl's Workout Prescription*. So many times a patient comes to see me, and I have the urge to write "exercise" on my prescription pad. Raising your fitness level is smart medicine. Some experts have been researching this for years and drawn the same conclusion. A large study in the journal *Epidemiology Research International*[1] quantified the effects of various health risks on the likelihood of dying for a group of 50,000 men and women. Low fitness stood out as the biggest predictor of death, more powerful even than smoking, obesity, diabetes, high cholesterol, and high blood pressure.

Think about that for a moment.

That means that if you're a middle-aged, obese smoker with high blood pressure, high cholesterol, and diabetes, the single best thing you can do to improve your health is exercise.

There's more. Researchers have looked at the relationship between exercise and many different types of health problems and overwhelmingly found that regular workouts—raising your fitness level—combat them all. That's a pretty compelling case for exercise.

Any health care practitioner worth his or her salt will tell you that it's always cheaper and easier to avoid illness than it is to treat it. Unfortunately, our current health care system is much more concerned with treating and managing disease than it is with prevention—which may be part of why we spend so much on health care (upwards of $300 billion annually on prescription medications alone) and yet have worse health outcomes than many countries that spend less.

My previous book, *The Exercise Cure*, goes into far more depth on this subject than I will here, but it's safe to say that we were made to move, and our bodies—virtually every cell from our brains to our toes—respond in wildly positive ways when we do. The problem is that too many of us don't.

Well, this is your friendly neighborhood drug dealer speaking: Exercise is medicine, and it's time for your fix! If all of this information isn't enough to convince you, like the infomercial says: But wait! There's more!

## Thinking about Skipping a Workout?

Research has shown that exercise is good medicine for the following problems: Obesity. High blood pressure. High cholesterol. Depression. Anxiety disorders. Dementia. Low self-esteem. Low energy.

Lower-back pain. Lousy sleep. Chronic fatigue. Asthma and allergies. Low libido. Erectile dysfunction. Premenstrual syndrome. Menopause symptoms. Osteoarthritis. Osteoporosis. Cognitive problems. Heart disease. Stroke. Type 2 diabetes. Metabolic disorder. Insulin resistance. Low immunity. Chronic pain.

It has also recently been shown to help prevent 17 types of cancer.

# Is Exercise Better Than "Real" Medicine?

I'm up-front about the therapeutic properties of exercise. But I want to be clear: Just because you exercise regularly, "real" medicine (in the form of procedures, pills, or any other method used to treat illness and injury) should never be ignored or avoided if you have a health problem. If you're sick or hurt, seek help. That's just common sense.

That said, I get this question all the time: "Is exercise better than 'real' medicine?" The answer is, "It depends." If you're having a heart attack as we speak, obviously you need an ER, not a gym. But after you have been treated and have recovered enough to be cleared by your doctor, exercise is crucial medicine both to help you fully recover and to prevent another heart attack.

Another example: Many health conditions, from type 2 diabetes to high cholesterol and high blood pressure, require medication. However, regular exercise could help improve these conditions to the point where meds may no longer be necessary—but only if your doctor sees enough improvement to warrant it.

My point is, a medical problem sometimes requires several methods of treatment. But exercise, in some instances, can gradually reduce the number of methods necessary until the only treatment you need is exercise itself.

That's the miracle drug at work.

## CAN EXERCISE KEEP YOU FROM AGING?

In 2009, three researchers—Elizabeth Blackburn, PhD; Carol Greider, PhD; and Jack Szostak, PhD—were awarded the Nobel Prize in Physiology or Medicine. Their discovery? How certain structures in our cells determine the rate at which we age.

By now, you may have heard the word *telomere*. Go deep into the nucleus of one of your cells. There you'll find your DNA, the blueprint of you. The DNA holds your chromosomes, which are long strings of genetic data. Telomeres protect the ends of your chromosomes, which would be damaged otherwise by cellular activity. The most common analogy you'll hear is that they are like plastic tips on the ends of your shoelaces.

Now, you know from Biology 101 that cells divide. What you may not know is that cells have a limited number of divisions in them. When you're young, your telomeres are long. Each time a cell divides, its telomeres shorten. If they get short enough, the cell will stop dividing and die. This process is called senescence. A senescent cell dies. So back to the shoelaces: Those plastic tips wear out and the shoelace frays. This is the biological aging process, although every person's telomeres shorten at different rates. Some folks age faster than others. Some folks get sick, which is both a sign of and a cause of telomere shortening. Not surprisingly, lifestyle plays a big role there. In a review of 27 studies published in *Circulation*,[2] shortened leukocyte (white blood cell) telomere length had a "significant association" with stroke, heart attack, and type 2 diabetes.

Telomeres have been studied for decades, but the 2009 Nobel discovery has truly broken open the floodgates of new research. And why not? It's possible that by achieving full understanding of telomeric aging and how to control it, we humans will have found our Fountain of Youth.

But let's not get ahead of ourselves. There are a few more things you need to know.

Telomeres didn't appear on the ends of your chromosomes out of thin air. At some point in our evolution, our cells determined the need for telomeres. In response, our bodies produced an enzyme called telomerase that produces and strengthens the telomeres. If you have good telomerase production, your telomeres will be longer.

Now, here's the interesting thing about all that research that's been going on: Some of it has focused on exercise and its potential effect on telomeres and telomerase—with a particular focus on HIIT and strength training. Consider: One 2008 study in *Archives of Internal Medicine*[3] observed 2,401 twins and found that the ones with increased physical activity levels had longer leukocyte telomeres than those who were less active. A sedentary lifestyle, the researchers concluded, may accelerate the aging process.

Another study, in *Medicine and Science in Sports and Exercise*[4] in 2015, looked at US data in regard to four types of "movement-based behavior" (that's a five-dollar term for *exercise*), moderate-intensity, vigorous-intensity, walking/cycling for transportation, and muscle-strengthening activity. Compared with participants who performed no exercise,

each group had lower odds of being in the bottom percentile for telomere length. However, the strength-training group had the best results by far.

A small 2016 study took a look not just at telomere length but also at telomerase activity. Researchers found that high-intensity interval running may increase telomerase in cells, resulting in longer telomeres.[5] (Previous research found similar results.)

Experts have also looked at the aging effects of exercise on older people. Two studies—one in the journal *Age*[6] and another in *PLOS ONE*[7]—analyzed the activities of adults ranging in age from 61 to 85. Both found that the greatest telomere benefits came to the people who exercised at the highest intensity.

And finally, a smaller 2014 study[8] recruited 21 healthy women in their twenties. One group went through a program of three HIIT running sessions per week for 8 weeks. The other group didn't change their behavior. The HIIT group, not surprisingly, showed "significant" telomere length, compared with the control group—as well as lower weight and body-fat percentage.

You know why I find this so interesting? As I mentioned earlier, it's so easy for people's expectations to get wrapped up in a number on the scale or how they might look in the mirror after exercising for a few weeks. But you can't see your cells in a mirror, and regular HIIT sessions have been shown time and again to have positive effects on your very DNA.

Is exercise the Fountain of Youth? Well, let me put it this way: The benefits are there. You may not be able to see them, but your body will experience them. Your body knows.

## THIS IS YOUR BRAIN ON EXERCISE

You didn't think we'd stop at your DNA, did you? As with studies on telomeres, research on how exercise affects your brain has gone in some interesting directions over the past few years. And again, science shows us that our lifestyle choices have an incredible impact on health and longevity. That statement may sound obvious, but what's surprising is how it happens.

Your brain, it turns out, behaves an awful lot like a muscle. If you have a sedentary lifestyle that includes other bad habits, your brain tends to shrink, just like a dormant muscle would atrophy. One particularly vulnerable area of the brain—and usually the first to suffer from a poor lifestyle or illness—involves the hippocampi, two seahorse-shaped nodes about the size of your thumb on the undersides of each brain hemisphere. The hippocampi are primarily responsible for short-term memory and consolidating it for long-term storage, which is why memory loss is one of the first symptoms of cognitive decline: Your hippocampi and short-term memory seem to go first. In the normal aging process the hippocampi generally shrink about 0.5 percent per year starting at age 50. The smaller your hippocampi, the more vulnerable you are to cognitive decline and dementia later in life.

What hurts the hippocampi? The list is not surprising: A 2012 study in *Nature Reviews Neurology*[9] found that the hippocampi are particularly vulnerable to the "neurotoxic" effects of obesity and its potential side effects, such as high blood pressure, obstructive sleep apnea, and type 2 diabetes. Some illnesses like depression and bipolar disorder may also contribute. According to the study, people with these conditions often have smaller hippocampi and experience greater cognitive decline than healthier individuals.

Now here's the interesting part: The hippocampi appear to respond to positive lifestyle choices just like a muscle would—as in, you can make them grow. The creation of new neurons in the brain is called *neurogenesis*. It's common sense: Create fresh neurons and the brain will grow and function better. And here's another term: *angiogenesis*. That's the creation of new blood vessels in the body, and yes, this can occur in the brain. New blood vessels mean better circulation in the brain, which means more oxygen feeding all those little gray cells. In short, neurogenesis and angiogenesis are very good for your brain. You want them to happen. Happily, they can happen at any age.

Now, would you be surprised to learn that exercise seems to promote both of these things?[10]

A 2014 study[11] tested participants with a single bout of resistance exercise (aka strength training) and found they had improved episodic memory performance up to 48 hours later, compared with those who didn't exercise. A *PLOS ONE* study[12] looked at 88 older adults; the ones who engaged in varying levels of physical activity, ranging from low to vigorous intensity, had healthier tissue in their temporal and hippocampal areas. Even walking may help neurogenesis: In another study,[13] in which participants expanded their walking sessions from 10 to 40 minutes, they grew their hippocampal volume by 2 percent in just 1 year. Researchers equate that to turning back the brain clock 2 to 4 years.

How does exercise work so much magic? Part of the equation could be bloodflow—a well-fed brain tends to be healthier. Also, brain experts speculate that exercise may promote the production of brain-derived neurotrophic factor (BDNF), a protein that acts as a fertilizer to brain cells.

There's one last thing I want to mention about a healthy brain. The research is still preliminary on this, but the concept of "cognitive reserve" looks very interesting going forward, especially as we all age. Cognitive reserve simply means you have brain to spare—one example would be your hippocampi being larger and healthier than in other folks the same age. Now researchers are discovering that having a good cognitive reserve may allow your brain to function normally as you age, even when the plaques and tangles that indicate dementia (and Alzheimer's disease in particular) are present. Doctors speculate that having a good cognitive reserve can allow the brain to perform a "self-bypass" around the unhealthy tissue. One very interesting study[14] examined elderly patients while they were alive and also postmortem and found that the one-third of the group with larger hippocampal volume indeed had plaques and tangles indicating dementia pathology yet had displayed no symptoms in life.

Did I mention that exercise helps grow your brain?

## FITNESS: A NEW CLASSIFICATION

If you visit your doctor, whether it's for an illness or a well visit, the staff will check your weight and blood pressure, listen to your heart and lungs, and ask you about your smoking habits. You know what they won't check? Your fitness level—despite all the research showing that low fitness is such a huge contributor to chronic illness.

I'm realistic about this. During the typical doctor's appointment, there's no time. And frankly, fitness is not a priority, especially if a patient has some pressing, immediate health concern. But it would be interesting to see health care pros administering fitness tests in exam rooms and hallways. Just ain't happenin'!

I'd like to make the argument that fitness is as important to a patient's medical profile as any other vital sign. In 2009, when the American College of Sports Medicine launched its "exercise is medicine" initiative, it included a statement encouraging medical professionals to consider physical activity and fitness level to be a vital sign to be checked during every patient visit—same as blood pressure, heart rate, and pupil response would be during an annual physical—and also to counsel patients about their physical activity and health needs, thus leading to overall improvement in the public's health and long-term reduction in health care costs.

I'm all on board for this (to no one's surprise, I'm sure!). The fact is that we simply don't give prevention its due. I do my best to emphasize exercise as medicine (particularly preventive medicine) with my patients and to impart smart exercise habits to the people who attend my weekly exercise classes. But I'm just one doctor. Given how important prevention is for both the individual and society at large, we should be offering more incentives for people to stay healthy.

I hope I'm offering you the biggest incentive of all right here: scientific proof of how amazing regular exercise is for your health and longevity. Knowledge is power (but as you'll see in Chapter 6, knowledge isn't always the key to inspiration; you'll find the secrets to true motivation there). Meanwhile, in my office, I want to help all the patients who come in, whether they walk, hop, limp, or use crutches. They've come for answers about the best ways to heal. I want to be able to offer patients clear directives that will not just get them through their injury or illness but also make the rest of their lives easier and more comfortable. I imagine many other doctors feel the same way. So it's not the easiest thing—or the most natural thing—for me to look a patient in the eye and say, "A lot of this is up to you."

Unfortunately, that's true. *No one has more power over your health than you.* It's all in your hands. Your doctor may not consider fitness to be a vital sign, but that shouldn't stop you from shooting for it. You can monitor this vital sign. You can maintain it. You can improve it. (See Chapter 5 for ways to measure your fitness.)

Now, I'm not ready to hang up my stethoscope and tell you that exercise is the cure for everything that ails you. Of course, real maladies require real medicine in the form of diagnosis, treatment, medication, and other interventions like surgery. What I hope I've made clear in this chapter, though, is that any exercise philosophy requires big-picture thinking that goes beyond the mirror and your bathroom scale. If you have a health problem, major or minor—or if you want to make sure health issues don't come looking for you—the first and simplest solution is to get moving.

To find out the best ways to do just that, keep on reading.

## CHAPTER THREE

# STEP 3: IT'S NOT ABOUT ABS OR A FIRM BUTT

## (But You Could Have It All!)

**Rock-Hard Abs!**

**Toned, Sexy Arms!**

**Your Best Butt Ever!**

Do any of those promises sound familiar? If you've ever stood in line at the grocery store and read the headlines on health and fitness magazines—you know, the kind full of guys with shredded torsos and celebrities in sexy bikinis—they should. Well, it's easy to make fun of these claims, but instead, let's analyze them.

That these magazines and photos exist means that a large group of average humans out there want what the headlines promise: the six-pack, the world-class butt, etc. That desire, at its most basic level, is pretty normal and can be a huge positive—if it motivates a person to exercise more.

Ever seen the movie *The Devil's Advocate*? In it, Al Pacino plays Satan himself, and one of his oft-repeated lines is "Vanity . . . my favorite sin." Well, if you look at those headlines, each one is specific to what the fitness industry refers to as vanity muscles, meaning the muscles that people (supposedly) want most and—let's be honest—the muscles

that we hope to have because they'll bring us the most attention; hence, the vanity.

But if vanity motivates people to take better care of themselves, to exercise more, to set and pursue a goal, is that bad? Of course not. When you consider how unhealthy a sedentary lifestyle is (and you just found out all about that in the previous chapter), anything that gets people moving consistently seems to me to be a good thing. Vanity can also be tied to higher self-esteem. A simple *Hey, my butt's looking pretty good lately!* can make you walk with more confidence, improve your mood, and push you to keep doing the good things you've been doing.

But there's major downside potential here: An excess of self-esteem isn't exactly an attractive trait. And training to make your vanity muscles "pop" can tempt you to train incorrectly—like doing endless crunches to tease out that six-pack, which could make you ignore other muscle groups to your body's detriment.

All of this goes back to what I said at the beginning: *You're not thinking big enough,* especially if you're training for a specific "magazine cover" body goal (better abs, arms, butt).

A simple shift in that thinking could change something good you're doing into something great.

## EVERYONE IS CREATED EQUAL (SORT OF)

Aside from the fact that chasing vanity muscles could make you exercise more, the end result will probably disappoint you. Here are some thoughts that might put it all into perspective.

- Not everyone is built to look the same way. But everyone is built to execute the same movements.

- Everyone has a set of rectus abdominis muscles to help his or her core function properly. But not everyone can grow a six-pack.

- Everyone has a set of gluteus muscles to help him or her run and jump and squat. But not everyone can have the butt of (name your celebrity).

Why are these things true? Some of it is genetics. Some people have different body types. Some people, let's be honest, simply don't look as "perfect" as others.

Here's the thing, and this is a big thing: *Everyone does have the same set of muscles. Everyone can train those muscles. That means that we can all build our own best body*—a body that propels us forward each day and helps us perform, stay active, work hard, have fun, break a sweat, keep healthy, and yes, look our best.

This is what I mean when I say that people don't always look at or think about the big picture when it comes to exercise.

Oh, and by the way, if you are truly motivated to exercise because you want those vanity muscles to pop? Training to build your best body—by definition—means that if you're destined to have a six-pack or world-class butt, you probably will. But if not? You'll still be living in your best body, with head-to-toe fitness, balanced muscle groups, and a physical capability that most people dream of but never achieve.

That sounds so much better to me than doing a lot of crunches or biceps curls.

## WHAT IS YOUR "BEST BODY"?

I've had some revelations over the years, incredible things that they never mentioned in medical school. Keep livin', keep learnin'! One of these things is how to more effectively train the human body. We know so much more now about how all of our mechanical parts interact, how an imbalance in one area can affect performance in another. Here's an example from my own experience: If you have a severe joint injury, your chances of developing osteoarthritis in that joint later in life go up. It's just the way it is. I blew out my knee in medical school, so yes, I have some arthritis in there. I don't want my triathlon training to be affected by this, let alone my day-to-day life—especially as I get older. Now, if I had just gone forward with all my endurance training without thinking about my knee—just powering through any discomfort—I'd have been setting myself up for real problems later on. But like I said, I've learned a few things. When I started strength training, my body got stronger, and my knee pain lessened.

I found I was able to do more and train harder. I'm still able to put a remarkable number of miles on my arthritic knee.

It was a beautiful thing: I could control my knee pain with strength.

Why? Muscle supports and stabilizes a joint. It's intuitive, but people don't always make the connection or think about how important this relationship is. It's not just the muscles close to the joint. My hips, glutes, and legs work together to keep the bones in my knee from grinding together. If you've ever experienced another common ailment—lower-back pain—the same concept applies: Your core and glute muscles help support your spine so nerves aren't compressed, sending you into spasm. Like the song says, the thighbone's connected to the hip bone (singing about femurs and pelvises isn't as catchy, I guess). Same goes for your muscles, tendons, and ligaments, as well as the fascia running through your muscles and the cartilage between all those bones. They're all connected, all working together to keep you strong, moving, and pain-free.

All of this interrelates with what I define as your "best body": well trained and in muscular balance from head to toe. Mobile. Flexible. Prepared for real-world tests. Resistant to injury. And, to an extent, resistant to illness.

I know, I know—not quite as sexy as six-pack abs but a million times more important, useful, and healthy. I train to achieve my best body, a body that will never be mistaken for a superhero's but one that allows me to do the things I want to do, on demand, in the real world. You'll never get there if you pursue the vanity muscles—tons of crunches for abs or curls for those biceps—because you'll be ignoring total-body training.

Total body leads to best body.

And now I'll show you the key to unlocking all that potential.

## YOUR BEST BODY VERSUS THE REAL WORLD

Picture yourself walking down the sidewalk. Easy, right? Just cruising along, legs moving, arms swinging. When you walk, you don't think about it. Well, today, let's think about it.

How many muscles are in the human body? It's hard to count, actually, and different experts will tell you different things. But there are (approximately, maybe, possibly) 650 skeletal muscles in the body. Some might say fewer; some, more. And that's just skeletal muscles that govern voluntary movement—not involuntary muscles that pump blood (you know which one I mean), move food through your GI tract, or give you goose bumps. So the scientific answer is . . . a lot.

How many muscles does it take to walk? A nice stroll feels effortless, so while it might not feel like many muscles, if you take your body in sections—feet, legs, hips, core, arms—well, that's a bunch of muscles, all working in concert just to move you down the sidewalk. One way to get some perspective: Imagine you had to build a humanlike cyborg that could walk, run, lift, or do anything a person can. You'd have to take into consideration all those moving parts just to get started. Walking: the simplest thing, until you analyze what's involved on a biomechanical level.

Now imagine jogging. Sprinting. Lifting grocery bags. Stuffing a carry-on into an overhead bin. Going in for a layup in a pickup basketball game or leaping to catch a Frisbee.

Each a symphony of movement. And all of these movements are made possible by the interconnected system of muscles, ligaments, tendons, bones, and so on called the kinetic chain. If you understand the concept of the kinetic chain—and if you "train the chain" instead of focusing on one body part or muscle group—you're working to create your very best body.

That, to me, is the single biggest piece of information you need when deciding to add total-body strength training to your life.

If you remember high school science class, *kinetic* relates to "motion or movement." So the kinetic chain is, at its most basic, a chain of movement—all those body parts working together to let you do all the things you do: each body part a link, each link depending on the others for normal, healthy movement— and abnormal, unhealthy movement, now that I think about it. (You don't want to slip on ice and fall, but if you do, look, kids, that's the kinetic chain in action!)

Now, knowing that I'm a sports medicine specialist, you might guess where I'm headed with all this. If all those muscles and other goodies form a head-to-toe chain, and a healthy chain leads to balanced movement, what happens around a weak link? Just what you'd think: injury. Wherever that weakness is, it will force other parts of the chain to compensate, which will lead to poor mechanics, and eventually something will give way. I see this in the majority of my patients: "I thought I might have tendinitis in my knee, but now my back hurts."

It's all connected, folks. So let's look more closely at how this chain really works. (And FYI, if you want to dig deeper, the back side of your body is the posterior chain; the front, the anterior. Then there are "open-chain" and "closed-chain" exercises. We could get far more technical, but I'm going to stick with the full-body approach for simplicity.)

First, I'll show you something about your body's movement mechanics that you may not know. Then we'll look at interaction up the chain. Keep in mind: All of this is geared toward giving you a working knowledge of your body so that when the time comes to start the workouts, you'll better understand how they are geared toward total-body, full-chain training.

## THE GENIUS OF JOINTS

Let's forget for a moment that part of the last chapter where I said I was a drug dealer, and let's talk about the kinds of joints that help you move (as opposed to the ones that make you lie on the couch and get the munchies). It's human nature to take things for granted, so you've probably never given much thought to how your joints work—not individually, which was covered in health class, but as a system. Read the following list of joints and their primary functions, starting from your toes to your head.

- Toes: stability

- Ankles: motion

- Knees: stability

- Hips: motion

- Spine: stability

- Shoulders: motion

- Elbows: stability
- Wrists: motion
- Knuckles: stability

Do you see the pattern? The joints alternate between stability and motion. Hinge joints like the elbow and knuckle offer stability to the joints that have freer movement, like the ankle and shoulder (but keep in mind that the spine is a very complex, very different animal from all the others).

Now, if your movements are normal and natural, you and your joints tend to get along just fine. If your movements go against that dynamic? Well, how about the knee? It's designed for stability. What happens if you ask it to become a motion joint? Ouch! How about the spine? If you use proper form, you can deadlift your body weight (or a lot more if you lift regularly) and all will be well. Twist the wrong way or lift something with lousy form and you just might find yourself bent over, holding your lower back and cursing yourself for the next 2 weeks.

And let's not forget: The space between all of these joints is occupied by a brilliant system of interconnected tissue like muscle, tendon, ligament, cartilage, blood vessels, and nerves. If you respect how all these pieces work together and train your chain with a brain, as it were, you're going to get better results and also prevent injury.

## Be a Coiled Spring

I love plyometric exercises as part of a complete exercise regimen. If you're not familiar with this term, *plyometrics* refers to exercises with explosive movement. Do them consistently and they can turn your body into a coiled spring. Everyone has two types of muscle fibers, fast twitch (used for sprinting and the aforementioned explosive movement) and slow twitch (used for longer-distance and endurance exercise). Every person has a different ratio of fast-twitch to slow-twitch fibers, thanks to just plain old genetics. That's part of the reason why parents who are successful distance runners breed good distance runners, while parents who are sprinters tend to breed sprinters. Explosive sports favor fast-twitch fibers, while endurance sports favor slow-twitch fibers. But the key to training is to make sure you're working both types. This is particularly important for the endurance sport athletes who forget about their fast-twitch muscles. Even if you run long distances exclusively or have a passion for endurance events, you still need to maintain a balance between fast- and slow-twitch muscles. This gives you more athletic ability, prevents overuse injuries, and keeps your body from becoming a one-trick pony.

Some examples of plyometric exercises are squat jumps, lunges, skater plyos (which mimic the side-to-side motion of speed skating), and compound movements like burpees (from standing, squat, thrust your legs back into a pushup position, do a pushup, return to squat position, then jump explosively—and repeat until you can't walk!). You'll find a set of plyometric workouts in this book (see page 158). Have some fun with them—they add an extra dimension to your strength training.

## Ever Go Barefoot?

Barefoot running became a big trend a few years back. It's not for everyone, but those who love it swear by it. I'm not going to suggest you try it—though if you want to, by all means do!—but I am going to suggest trying barefoot strength workouts.

They can really give your feet an extra kick, as it were.

To start, I suggest doing a short workout—10 minutes is good, and the workouts in this book are divvied up that way—on a surface that gives you some cushion, like carpeting in your home. As your feet become stronger, graduate to longer barefoot workouts.

The beach is also good for barefoot training. If no beach is available, how about your lawn? Keepin' it interesting!

I'm going to go into some detail in this section, and that's deliberate. There's something important I want you to know, but I won't tell you what it is until after you read this section. Trust me, it's worth it!

To start, I'd like to show your feet some respect. Everything begins with the feet. They're the foundation of almost all movement. A foot is an amazing, dynamic structure, a collection of 26 bones, 33 joints, 19 muscles and tendons, and 107 ligaments housed in a space the size of a . . . well, a foot. Why so many moving parts? Your feet don't just have to support your body weight, they also need to propel it in different directions, sometimes with explosive force. Foot stability is essential to healthy movement.

Every single exercise in my HIIT workouts involves the feet in some way, so your foundation will get its share of play as we intrinsically train all the muscles in each foot. That's a good thing: Those muscles are responsible for supporting all the bones in the foot, and people can develop weak foot muscles simply from wearing supportive shoes all the time—not to mention all the sitting we do nowa-days. So respect your feet and they'll get you where you're going in style.

How do your feet interact with the rest of the kinetic chain? There's a strong connection between foot mechanics and knee position, so when you walk or run, for example, your leg and knee can be affected by how your foot strikes the ground. Some people pronate, which means their foot turns inward as it strikes. Other people supinate, which means their foot turns outward as it strikes. Some fortunate and/or well-trained runners have a neutral foot strike, which is the healthiest for the rest of your body.

Here's how this applies to you: If your foot rolls in, you put a lot more stress on the inside part of the shin. Shin splints are often related to a foot that rolls in too much. Plus, the most common knee pain we see in the office, patellofemoral knee pain (pain under the kneecap), happens oftentimes because the foot rolls in too much. But here's another kinetic chain reaction: This knee pain can also be caused by weak muscles in the hips and pelvis. That's right, you can have a knee injury caused by either your foot strike or your hip strength.

The knee has the distinction of being caught between the ground and the hip, sandwiched in between. Links in a chain that depend on each other, folks!

## HOW THESE LINKS CLICK

Hopefully, you're beginning to understand how your body moves. Muscle function is very much related to joint function and vice versa. That's why I'm such a huge proponent of total-body training, building all your muscles so your kinetic chain works better. As you'll see, the workout section of the book is loaded with exercises that hit as many muscles and joints as possible in a short time, to be performed at high repetition and high intensity—whatever your personal pace may be to achieve that result.

But back to the chain: Moving up past the knees, we arrive at one of the most complex interconnected sections. Everything from your quads and hamstrings up into your hips and glutes and then your core—particularly your back—works together, and yet here's where people tend to neglect one part to the detriment of the whole family. Think of all the potential injuries: back pain, strained groin, hamstring pull, etc. Back pain is a big-gie—four out of five adults experience it at some point. Back pain can be caused by a specific back injury, such as a herniated disc. But the back muscles are also tied deeply into the kinetic chain, which means that back pain is interrelated with hamstring flexibility, hip flexor tightness, and core strength. The dreaded "back spasms" can be exacerbated by imbalances in any or all of these areas. If you work to stay strong and flexible in your hammies and hips and hit your core hard (I love planks for core stability—and of course the book has a core workout series; see page 238), you'll greatly reduce the compressive forces around the back joints.

Which leads us to your shoulders, a pair of ball-and-socket joints and the least stable ones in the body. Your shoulder is very susceptible to muscular forces behind and in front of the joint. The good news? The shoulder is also the most susceptible joint to strengthening. Weak muscles can create a lot of problems for swimmers, rowers, or anyone who performs an overhead movement that puts a lot of demand on the shoulders (that could be spiking a volleyball or trying to stuff that way-too-fat carry-on into the overhead bin; just check it, dude!). Strong muscles stabilize the shoulder joint and can prevent a host of problems.

## Try One at a Time

To really give your lower body a workout, try a couple sets of single-leg exercises. I've suggested this to some of my patients who needed to get their lower halves in better shape, and they've reported good results. Try single-leg squats (a real challenge!), single-leg hops, and lunges with the rear foot elevated, movements where you use your own body weight but also have to balance. That balancing act is huge. It gets all those small supporting muscles around the joints to fire. You should notice greater strength and stability around your ankles, knees, and hips in short order.

## The Important Part

Why did I want you to read all that? Simple. I want you to have an awareness of how the entire body functions as a cohesive unit. I want you to have images in your mind. I want you to be able to imagine, acknowledge, and feel your body as it moves, particularly when you exercise. This isn't just so you can appreciate what your body can do, though that's part of it. This total-body awareness allows you to focus on proper muscle engagement, form, and follow-through. That kind of mindfulness toward each exercise will make you perform it better, which makes bad training habits easier to break (one of the worst is rushing a movement to raise your rep count). This also leads to more athleticism and better overall results in the long run.

Now let's take a look at another kinetic chain issue and something that confuses and frustrates a lot of people.

## "HOW CAN I BE MORE FLEXIBLE?"

I get that question a lot. And I understand why people ask it. But I wish they'd ask it in a different way: "What does *flexibility* really mean?"

Now that's a good question.

When people think of flexibility, they think of the human epitome of it: the ballet dancer, the gymnast, the circus contortionist. Honestly, these are not realistic models to have in mind when it comes to your own twisting and stretching. In the context of our goal—training for total-body fitness—improved flexibility is a component but not the overall goal. The technical definition of *flexibility* is "a muscle's ability to extend over its full range." Most people, however, can do well with this definition: "an ability to perform daily tasks and movements without undue tightness, pain, or injury."

Notice that I say "undue." If you have to suddenly bend down or reach high, you might feel a twinge. That's normal. But to assign a uniform set of flexibility goals to every person is unrealistic. Some people can touch their toes effortlessly. Others never will, and somehow these people will still lead long and productive lives. So how do we set goals for improved flexibility that anyone can pursue successfully?

First, I don't think it's a stretch (sorry) to say that most people, even those who are generally fit, aren't very flexible. Your joints may feel tight and creaky, your muscles and connective tissue wound tight; twisting or bending your spine in any direction may feel challenging or unpleasant. This isn't an injury per se, but it's a physical issue that could lead to injury—and it definitely holds you back in any activity.

What causes this? If a muscle is short or tense, its full range will be limited. Ditto if the fascia, a tough tissue that wraps around and weaves through the muscles, or the tendons, which attach the muscles to your bones, are short or tight. Injury, inactivity, poor posture, poorly coordinated movement, and genetics—how flexible your parents are—can directly affect the length of these tissues. From what I see in my practice, sitting has become the biggest enemy of flexibility.

Tension in your muscles is another big factor. Most muscles have some degree of tension—or tonus—in them all the time, even when you feel relaxed. Muscle tension can be affected by injury, stress, heavy work, or hard exercise, and by repetitive movements with a small range of motion. DOMS—delayed-onset muscle soreness, which can come on 12 to 48 hours following a hard workout—can also cause stiffening and tightness in the muscles.

One good reason to pay attention to your flexibility? Over time, tight muscles can become more than a minor inconvenience. One inflexible muscle group can eventually cause muscle groups on the opposite side of a joint to stop working altogether. As that muscle group sits on the sideline, still other muscles have to step in and pick up the slack. This domino effect can eventually cause even the most basic movement pattern—like walking or driving—to become uncoordinated and painful.

I'll paint you a picture: When the muscles in the hip flexor group on the fronts of your hips become short—a common consequence of sitting—the front of your pelvis gets pulled forward and down when you stand. Your lower back then has to work extra hard to pull you upright, and the biggest muscles in your body—your glutes—suddenly have a hard time doing their job. A host of problems can result: back pain, tight hamstrings, a rounded back, a head that protrudes forward, painful shoulders. Eventually, other problems related to poor movement, including sciatica, can develop. A similar cascade of problems can occur when the flexibility limitations occur in the upper back and neck.

Clearly, all of us need some amount of flexibility training to avoid pain and move comfortably through our everyday life.

The upshot? How flexible you are is largely

## Yoga: Are You Missing Out?

Old-school static stretching—"static" meaning you don't move while you do it (as in holding that hamstring stretch for 30 seconds)—isn't nearly as effective for total-body flexibility as regular yoga. (I'll even throw in Pilates classes as a bonus!) In yoga, you're learning to relax and be comfortable in fully extended, stretched positions. It delivers movement-based flexibility and can transform your body (Pilates also hammers your core). You'll feel more powerful, movement will be easier and more fluid, and, most important, you'll reduce your injury risk.

I think of strength HIIT and yoga as an amazing one-two total-body punch that can make you physically unstoppable.

based on the activities you do. If you add some activities that aid flexibility—the HIIT workouts do that, but you can do even more—your body will be better for it. So how much and what kind of flexibility training does the average person need?

The key with flexibility is not to see how far you can stretch but to keep all your moving parts in a more or less balanced relationship, so that nothing is either too tight or too loose. Again, you want to be able to perform any task without tightness or pain. You can see this in young children, who have yet to suffer acute injuries or develop overuse problems, and thus tend to have a good balance among muscle groups.

There are two stretching modalities I particularly like: dynamic stretching—which you can do anytime but should do before any workout—and yoga, which you can do on off days as part of your recovery process (see Chapter 7 for more). In dynamic stretching, you're essentially practicing athletic movement, and I'm a big fan of all things athletic.

## THE ART OF THE DYNAMIC STRETCH

These anywhere, anytime stretches are a terrific way to increase flexibility for everyday activities and sports alike. You'll see that these form a longer version of the Dynamic Warmup in the workout section. The difference is that here we have a couple more exercises and no timed HIIT format. Do these stretches at your own pace, and use them as a quick energy booster anytime throughout your day.

Directions: Move into each stretch at a deliberate speed, hold for 1 count, and then come out of it slowly. Repeat each stretch 5 to 10 times per side.

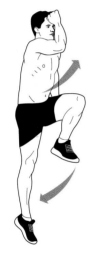

### HIGH KNEES

Stand tall with your feet shoulder-width apart. Without changing your posture, raise your left knee as high as you can and step forward. Repeat with your right knee. Continue to alternate back and forth while pumping your arms as if sprinting. (Note: In the workout section, High Knees are more of a sprint exercise.)

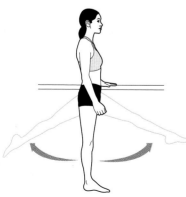

### HIP SWING

Stand tall and hold on to a sturdy object with your left hand. Brace your core. Keep your left knee straight, and swing your left leg forward as high as you comfortably can. Then swing your left leg backward as far as you can. That's 1 rep. Swing forward and back continuously. Complete all your reps, then do the same with your right leg.

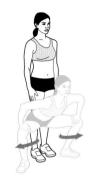

### GATE SWING

Stand with your feet together and your hands at your sides. Drop into a squat by pushing your hips back and lowering your body toward the floor, while keeping your back upright. As you lower yourself, hop your feet wider with your toes pointing outward, and gently press your hands into your inner thighs to facilitate the stretch. Hop back to the starting position and repeat.

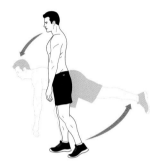

### SINGLE-LEG, STRAIGHT-LEG DEADLIFT REACH

Stand with your arms at your sides. Raise your left foot and left hand. Slowly lower your torso and touch the toes of your right foot with your left hand. Return to the starting position. Do all your reps on one side, then switch sides.

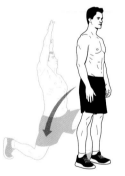

### REVERSE LUNGE AND REACHBACK

Stand tall with your feet hip-width apart. Step backward with your right leg, and lower your body until your left knee is bent at least 90 degrees. Once in this position, reach your arms up and back toward your left shoulder. Press back up to a standing position, and then step back with your left leg, this time reaching toward your right.

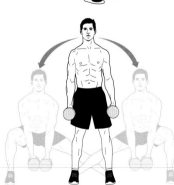

### LOW SIDE-TO-SIDE LUNGE

Stand with your feet shoulder-width apart and clasp your hands in front of your chest (or hold dumbbells, as illustrated). Shift your weight to your right leg and lower your body, bending your right knee and pushing your butt back. Keep your left leg straight and left foot flat on the floor. Without raising yourself all the way to standing, reverse the movement to the left. Alternate back and forth. Note: Be sure to push your hips back as you lower down and engage your core to keep your upper body vertical.

## FLOOR Y-T-I RAISES

Note: Do one set of 8 to 10 reps of each.

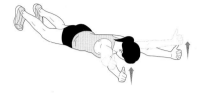

### Y RAISE

Lie facedown on the floor. Allow your arms to rest on the floor, stretching above your head, each arm completely straight and at a 30-degree angle to your body, palms facing each other and thumbs up. Your body should resemble the letter *Y*. Raise your arms as high as you can, pause, and then slowly lower back to the starting position.

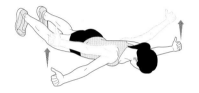

### T RAISE

Lie facedown on the floor. Move your arms so they're out to your sides, perpendicular to your body, with your thumbs pointing up. Your body should resemble the letter *T*. Raise your arms as high as you can. Pause, then slowly lower back to the starting position.

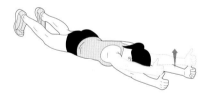

### I RAISE

Lie facedown on the floor. Position your arms straight above your shoulders so your body forms a straight line from your feet to your fingertips. Your palms should be facing each other, thumbs pointing up. Your body should resemble the letter *I*. Raise your arms as high as you can, pause, and then slowly lower back to the starting position.

### INCHWORM

Stand tall with your legs straight, and bend over and touch the floor. Keeping your legs straight, walk your hands forward. (If you can't reach the floor with your legs straight, bend your knees just enough so you can. As your flexibility improves, try to straighten them a little more.) Keeping your core braced, walk your hands out as far as you can without allowing your hips to sag.

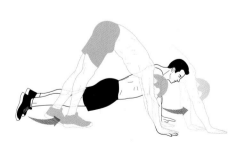

Then take tiny steps to walk your feet to your hands. That's 1 repetition. Do 3 forward, then 3 more in reverse.

## WHAT RATTLES YOUR CHAIN?

Okay, you've learned a lot about your kinetic chain so far. The HIIT workouts in this book will help train it in a balanced way. But I'm a sports doctor, so I want to not just help you build your body, I also want to help you avoid hurting it. Here are some of the most common scenarios that can bring on an injury.

- **Stress.** Not *I'm-stuck-in-traffic-kill-me-now* stress. I mean putting stress on a body part—muscle, ligament, joint, etc.—that is unprepared for it or can't handle it. This is common in former scholastic athletes, now sofa surfers who haven't done anything for a few years and fall prey to Too Syndrome (too much, too fast, too soon). It can also happen to well-conditioned athletes who simply move in a way their bodies disagree with. These kinds of injuries can be severe and even shocking. You think, *Whoa, I'm really hurt here*, but I guarantee you use much stronger language.

- **Imbalance.** Put simply, your body isn't properly trained for the activity you're doing. Someone who runs nothing but half-marathons for 5 years suddenly decides a 100-meter sprint is a good idea. Well, distance running trains your hamstrings in the exact opposite way of what's required for a sprint. Guess who's limping home? That's why I keep stressing total-body training. Switch up your activities and hit all muscle groups. Back in the Dark Ages when I was rehabbing my knee, I'd sit in the gym and do leg extensions and hamstring curls—isolated movements that have no basis in reality. Now I never use those machines. I do balance work, single-leg work, and plyometric exercises like lunges and squat jumps, real-world movements that hit a lot of muscles at the same time and keep the body in balance. If you neglect body parts that can throw your muscles out of balance, you're just asking for the pain.

- **Overuse.** This one is common sense and yet still so common. If you work your body too hard, it will break down. It's like any other machine that needs maintenance and restoration (see Chapter 7 for lots more on this). But if you don't listen to your body and know your limitations, you'll never know when to back off. Again, guess who's limping home?

My work here is done (but not really, just in this chapter—there's lots more coming). We've covered a lot of ground, run through lots of great information, and I hope you now have a much better sense of what exercise can really do for you. I keep stressing big-picture thinking when it comes to working out, and I hope I've convinced you. Now keep reading. There's more to learn—and I'd like to formally give you my Exercise Prescription. Time for the miracle drug to do its work!

## CHAPTER FOUR

# YOUR EXERCISE PRESCRIPTION

By now, you've absorbed a lot of important information about exercise. Before we move on to the next section of the book, I want to take a quick breather so you have time to let it all sink in. I hope I've convinced you of a few important things.

**A.** Thinking about a bigger picture when it comes to exercise—and what you want to get out of it—will change your workout philosophy in a wonderful way. It's okay to want a "hotter body" or to "look great naked." It's also okay to want to get better at (insert your athletic goal here). But I believe you'll get better results—and achieve those other goals, too—if you consider the factors I mentioned in the first three chapters and adopt them all as a new exercise philosophy. Thinking about that bigger picture will mean fewer skipped workouts, deeper thought about what exercise means as an activity and a life asset, and a more focused mind when it's time to put on those sneakers.

**B.** HIIT workouts are worth the effort. They're time efficient and intense, and they deliver incredible results. Start with one

10-minute workout from these pages and keep going. Your body will thank you.

**C.** Exercise is medicine. You can build a body that's resistant to illness and injury. You can improve and perhaps eliminate conditions you already have. Health and longevity may not be sexy, hot-button subjects, but regular workouts can keep you mobile and smiling well into your later years. (And no matter how invincible you think you are now, trust me. Just trust me. And thank me later!)

**D.** Total-body strength training can cure muscle imbalances, prevent injury, and improve overall physical performance— whether your favorite activity is running or gardening, basketball or dancing. If you eliminate weak links in your kinetic chain, you will have created your best body.

Okay, that's enough philosophy class for now. Before we move on, I want to give you my comprehensive Exercise Prescription. It's easy for me to say, "Go forth and work out," but to get the most out of the prescription, you're going to need a few extra tips. I want this experience to be the most positive thing you've ever done, something that will last a (very long) lifetime. So here it is—your Exercise Prescription. Use it in good health!

**Exercise regularly and with purpose.** This is the obvious part of the prescription. If you're not breaking a sweat, you're not getting your optimal dose of the world's best medicine. All the benefits, all the goals, all the talk? Empty promises unless you're exercising. And when I say "with purpose," I mean that you should think about what you want out of it. That could be a goal like finishing a race or hitting a new fitness level. It could be about looking good for a class reunion or a new relationship or about fixing a health issue. That's up to you, and it's yours alone. But exercising is better when your mind and body are aligned for a single purpose. Get after it!

**Remember the big picture.** For some, exercise is a means to an end, but for me, it's meaningful and has no end. Movement is a part of life but also a gift. The more personal meaning you give to exercise—the privilege of movement—the more committed you'll be to it, and the more you'll enjoy it. Of all the positives of exercise I've already mentioned, here are some I haven't: Confidence. Satisfaction. Perspective. Those who consider the big picture take nothing for granted.

**Never sacrifice form for volume.** The HIIT workouts in this book are high volume, high intensity. But proper form is crucial, especially if you're just starting out. You may be tempted to go faster and skimp on full motion (I see way too many people doing "halfsie" pushups really fast to boost their rep count). Don't. When in doubt, slow down and savor the movement. Feel the muscles

engage, even during explosive movement. I'd rather you do 5 perfect reps than 15 lousy ones. Ignore form and, at best, your results will suffer. At worst, you'll hurt yourself.

**Go hard.** You want to be out of breath. You want to drip sweat. You want to feel the burn. You do *not* want to hurt yourself. You do *not* want to collapse. You do *not* want to vomit (you laugh, but some trainers think working so hard that you hurl is a good thing). That said . . .

**Keep going.** Never be afraid to push your limits.

**Seek upward.** Exercise isn't just the workout. It can become something more. Talk to fellow exercisers. Look for groups. Find a community. Maybe it's one person, maybe it's 20, maybe it's a social network a thousand strong. If you strive to seek the positive, to push to higher levels and bring others with you, all those simple little workouts can become transformative.

**Be flexible—to a point.** Life happens. Life is gravity. People and circumstances pull you in opposing directions. As much as you want your workout time to be nonnegotiable, sometimes you have to bargain. Sacrifice is not the end of the world. But you know what? You can also learn how to use the word *no* and have no regrets.

**Stop when it hurts.** An acute injury is darn well unmistakable. If you yank a hammie or hurt your knee or roll your ankle, you'll know it. That's not what I'm talking about. "The burn" is also obvious. It means you're challenging your muscles and good things will come of it. I'm not talking about that, either. I'm talking about the "almosts." The sensation you get when something feels like it's about to blow: a twinge in your lower back; a tug at the base of your glute; that other kind of burn on the bottom of your foot that's on the verge of full bloom. Folks, you don't want any of these things to actually bloom. It's definitely a subjective feeling, but if you sense anything like this, back off. Push your limits, not your luck.

**Accessorize.** Think about all the things you can add to your workout that will make it more fun and interesting. Music is a big one for a lot of people. Set up a playlist and change it up once a week. Or try a new radio app or a new music channel on your favorite music site. Another easy way to fuel the fire: Track your progress. I'll talk more about this in Chapter 5, but some people love tracking improvement. It gives you something to analyze daily, weekly, or monthly. And what about the swag? Fitness trackers, smartwatches, groovy water bottles, shoes, shirts, tank tops, and all manner of cool-looking gear can make you feel like conquering the world one rep at a time. If you're one of those people who love shopping for stuff, adopting

an exercise lifestyle opens up a whole new world of possibilities! This is a different form of shopping—and you have to train to make it happen—but I know many people who collect event T-shirts. It's a way of life, I'm tellin' ya.

And finally . . .

**Smile.** This is the most important part! Bring your positivity, your joy, your grin to every workout. I see far too many people who show up to workouts as if showing up for a daily root canal. Attitude really is everything. Is exercise a challenge? Of course. Does it make you work for it? Definitely. But let me tell you—from someone who has experienced far too many Mile 22s on the last leg of an Ironman triathlon—even when you're exhausted, even when it hurts, even when you don't think you can go 1 second more, the ability to call upon a smile as a secret weapon is the closest thing humans have to a superpower. Your smile—genuine and contagious to all around you—will be the difference. Today will be better because of your smile. You'll be back tomorrow because of your smile.

# PART TWO

# What Happens between Your Workouts

What happens *between* your workouts is more important than what happens *during* your workouts. Seriously. We're talking about some of the most critical physical activities and processes. This section will help you use that time to ensure that your body and mind are ready to achieve the best results possible. Sound like a lot of hard sell? Extra nonsense? Want to just plow ahead into the exercise section? Resist the temptation! The next three chapters will help you help yourself. Do you know how to evaluate your own fitness? Do you know what could be the most revealing fitness test of all? Do you know how to stay motivated? Do you know the secret to never skipping a workout? Do you know how to help your body bounce back from exercise? Do you know what is—no lie—the most important activity of your day? Here's a hint: It is *not* exercise.

Read on, and make everything better!

## CHAPTER FIVE

# THE DOCTOR'S 30-MINUTE FITNESS EVALUATOR

Here's what I like best about doing self-tests to measure fitness: You never get a wrong answer. The result is a snapshot in time, not a life sentence nor a mark on your permanent record. Whatever your result, you can build on it (or build in another direction). These tests reveal strengths and weaknesses, not final analyses. What you come up with today will be different from what you come up with a few weeks from now. Therein lies the usefulness: It's all about you, where you are, and where you can go.

A lot of people ask me, "How do I know if I'm fit?" The short answer is, "You can't." It's totally subjective and individual. That's what this chapter is all about: finding out where you are on your own fitness journey today. A month from now, after trying my HIIT workouts, you can test yourself again and see what's happened. I bet you'll be happy!

First, I want to give you a quick explanation of these DIY tests.

*What they are:* simple, fast ways to get an idea of certain fitness benchmarks. They give you a set of numbers you can use for comparison against later tests.

*What they aren't:* sophisticated evaluation tools. This is not the NFL Combine. Testing systems exist to reveal muscle imbalances and predict injury in elite competitive athletes (the Functional Movement Screen is one), but these tests are about measuring improvement, not parsing folders of data on your physical condition. If that's what you're looking for, I suggest . . . trying out for the Olympics?

Ultimately, what you're looking for here is a little bit of knowledge. An idea. *This is where I am right now.* Then use the prospect of another measurement in a month as motivation to improve: *How far can I go?*

I always dug that idea, so full of potential: *How far can I go?*

Let's find out.

## THE BEST FITNESS TEST OF ALL TIME

You didn't think we'd start slow, did you? I call this test the best because it reveals so much in such a short time. It's based on a Brazilian study[1] of 2,000 men and women, ages 51 to 80.

Here's how you do it: Sit down on the floor cross-legged. Now stand.

That's the test. So simple. What does it

# What's the Definition of *Fit*?

One definition of *fit* could be the ability to do whatever you want to do with your body (think gymnast). Another could be the ability to run great distances without stopping (think marathoner, though some folks might say even a 10K race is a long distance). Yet another could be the ability to sprint 40 yards while weighing 260 pounds to tackle someone (think linebacker). What about a pro tennis player? An Olympic pole vaulter? A biathlete able to cross-country ski and almost immediately steady her heart rate to shoot a rifle at a target with world-class marksmanship? Now, are all those people's fitness levels equal? Of course not. But all of them in their own way are fit.

A more useful question to ask yourself—and one that's easier to answer—is this: How should *I* define *fit*? You may have outsized expectations based on the definitions mentioned above. You may think someone who can do 25 pullups without stopping is "fit," but does that mean you need to do the same to achieve true fitness?

Set realistic, achievable goals. Hit them, then set slightly bigger, achievable goals. Repeat. Don't stop. And a funny thing will happen: Not only will you morph into an undeniable definition of *fit*, but your definition will change along with your fitness level—in the best way possible.

tell you? How fast you can get up and how much help you need gives a clear picture of your overall strength, flexibility, and coordination. Could you get up in only a few seconds without using your hands or any other assistance? That's a good sign of overall fitness. Did you need to use your hands to brace yourself on the floor? Did you need help from a wall or furniture or another person? Did it take you more than a few seconds? All those are signs of lower fitness—and in the study, the folks with the higher fitness lived longer. Now there's some incentive to stay fit.

My advice: Perform this test every 4 weeks as you exercise. See how much you improve!

### A Note for Beginners

It's common sense: If you haven't been exercising or you've been doing it for only a short time, the concept of a fitness test may intimidate you or, worse, seem pointless. *Not so, no way, no how.* I think these tests are crucial—especially if you've never done them before. These are your first steps, and they can be the most important for several reasons.

■ **You'll face your fear.** What else would make you hesitate to take these tests other than fear? But what are you afraid of? Failure? There's no pass/fail grade here. Embarrassment? If you take the tests by yourself, who's to know? Shame that you're not as fit as you want to be or as others around you or as people you see on TV? Well, improvement is the whole point of beginning an exercise regimen, isn't it? I say take pride in your first steps. You'll look back on them with a smile when you get where you're going.

- **You'll be forced to see reality.** Some folks think they're fitter than they really are. The tests don't sugarcoat it. If you feel frustration or shame at your results, think of those emotions as rocket fuel. It's not a failure. It's an opportunity. Take it!

- **You'll get a taste of the workouts.** Let's be honest: If you're just starting out, you may be out of shape, overweight, and hyperaware of those facts. Exercising for the first time—or after a long layoff—may be challenging, uncomfortable, and, as a result, intimidating. I'm asking you to put those thoughts aside. Do this battery honestly, without negativity or preconceived notions of what you think fitness is or should be. *Just start.* Get your results down on paper. Keep them to yourself if you like or share them for encouragement. But stay on the journey for 4 weeks and test yourself again.

I dare you to amaze yourself.

## Do You Have a Running Imbalance? Take the Test!

The workouts in this book are based on interval strength training, but I know two things: One, a lot of people enjoy running as a form of exercise, and it's a great activity for days you're not doing the HIIT workouts. Two, I run. A lot. I have a soft spot in my heart for an activity that's cheap and requires nothing more than tied shoes and miles (or a working treadmill). The understated answer: I encourage running. So I'd like to see everyone do it in a healthy way.

Proper form is important for running, just as much as it is for strength training. How do you know if you have a muscle imbalance that might be affecting your form? I have runners in my office do a simple step-down test, once for each leg. They step down off a small box or stool and I look at their pelvis straight on. The pelvic bones on either side—the bone points you can feel at the front of each hip—should aim straight ahead, completely level, like a car's headlights. That means you have good pelvic stability.

Usually what I see when a runner steps down is a hip sagging on one side, whichever side is weaker. This result almost always comes from the athlete not training the whole body. Too many times patients tell me they go to the gym and do leg extensions and hamstring curls, exercises that target one muscle apiece and don't address the kinetic chain. If you do that, you can end up with functional instability, which increases your injury risk. Paying attention to total-body conditioning can help correct any muscle imbalance.

To do this test at home: Set up a box or stool or anything that lets you step down about 18 inches to 2 feet. Set it up in front of a mirror, and slowly step down to the floor. Watch those pelvic bones as you do it, or have someone with a good eye watch them for you (recording this on a smartphone is a good idea). Do the step-down test once for each foot.

If one side of the hips sags? Add a set of single-leg exercises (squats, lunges, or hops) on that side to your regular workout to help reestablish balance. Retest yourself every week until you fix the imbalance.

## THE SIX-POINT DIY FITNESS BATTERY

That's a fancy name for the six exercises you'll do here. Each measures a certain aspect of fitness. As I mentioned, they aren't going to show up on ESPN highlight reels. They're quick and simple. You can run through the entire battery in a few minutes—however, I suggest giving yourself 3 to 4 minutes to rest between exercises. This isn't meant to be a circuit workout or, dare I say it, an interval set. You should be reasonably fresh for each new exercise.

Okay, here we go. This battery will measure, in no particular order, upper-body strength and mobility, core strength, lower-body strength and flexibility, balance and stability, and cardiovascular fitness.

Like I said, when you first try these tests, you may do well or you could struggle. It doesn't matter. What does matter is *how you improve over time*. If you follow the workouts

# If You Feel Pain . . .

These tests are designed to assess your current fitness levels. However, they could also reveal a hidden injury or problem. If at any time any of these movements causes you pain (which is not to be mistaken for "the burn" or fatigue), I advise you to see a physician or physical therapist to make sure that there's no underlying injury.

in this book, I know you'll see improvements. In theory, you could test yourself every week, but I suggest every 4 weeks. Ultimately, that's a random number, but once a month makes it easy to remember, and the results you see will be drastic enough to be meaningful.

Perform each of the exercises below in the order listed. Rest 3 to 4 minutes after each to make sure that you're not overly fatigued. After 4 weeks, have at it again and see how you do!

| EXERCISE | WEEK 1 NOTES | WEEK 4 NOTES |
|---|---|---|
| **Overhead Squat (10 reps)** | | |
| **Wall Slide (10 reps)** | | |
| **Plank (max time)** | | |
| **Pushup (1 minute)** | | |
| **One-Legged Balance Touch (1 minute, each leg)** | | |
| **300-Yard Shuttle Run** | | |

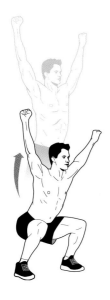

## OVERHEAD SQUAT

Fully extend your arms above your head, slightly more than shoulder-width apart. With your feet shoulder-width apart, lower your body as far as you can by pushing your hips back and bending your knees. Your torso should stay as upright as possible. Pause, then push yourself back up to the starting position. Perform 10 reps.

**WHAT IT TELLS YOU:** Watching yourself in a mirror helps answer the following questions.

- Can you lower your body until your thighs are below parallel to the floor? (Are your knees bent past 90 degrees?)
- Can you keep your heels on the floor?
- Can you keep your toes pointing straight ahead?
- Are your hands drifting forward as you squat and are your back and chest leaning forward?
- Do your knees cave inward?

Any of these problems could mean a variety of weaknesses, ranging from poor mobility in your upper and lower body to poor stabilization and control.

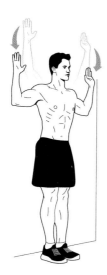

## WALL SLIDE

Stand with your head, upper back, and butt against a wall. Place both of your hands and arms against the wall in the "high-five" position, elbows bent 90 degrees and upper arms at shoulder height. Keeping your elbows, wrists, and hands against the wall, slide your elbows down toward your sides as far as you can. Squeeze your shoulder blades together as you go. Then slide your arms back up the wall as high as you can while keeping your hands in contact with the wall. Lower to the start and do 10 reps.

**WHAT IT TELLS YOU:**

- Do your elbows or hands come off the wall?
- How high can you slide your hands up the wall? Can you get them overhead?
- Do you feel any pain in your shoulders or upper back?
- Can you keep your shoulder blades squeezed together?

If you struggle with this exercise, it most likely means you need to improve your shoulder strength and flexibility.

## PLANK

Set a stopwatch and perform a plank for as long as you can.

**WHAT IT TELLS YOU:** This test assesses your core strength, including the strength of your abs, glutes, and lower back.

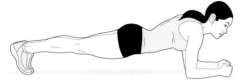

## PUSHUP

Do as many pushups as you can in 1 minute.

**WHAT IT TELLS YOU:** Pushups are a great assessment of upper-body strength and conditioning. They also rely on core strength and shoulder mobility, which will both be improved by our HIIT workouts.

## ONE-LEGGED BALANCE TOUCH

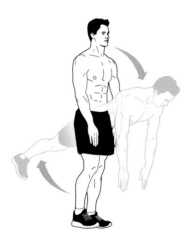

Set a timer for 1 minute. Stand with your legs shoulder-width apart. Lift your left foot about an inch off the floor, balancing on your right foot. Reach forward with your right hand, bending at the hip while keeping your left leg straight and extended out behind you, and touch the floor (you can use one hand or two). Return to the starting position and repeat as often as you can without breaking form for 1 minute. Repeat the process on your left leg.

**WHAT IT TELLS YOU:** How good is your balance, and how well do your legs help provide that balance? You should find out with this test. You should also be able to determine whether one leg is stronger or delivers better balance than the other.

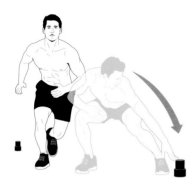

## 300-YARD SHUTTLE RUN

Pace off a 25-yard distance. Run the 25 yards, then return to where you started. Complete this 50-yard round-trip run six times, and record your time.

**WHAT IT TELLS YOU:** It's a marker for speed and conditioning—and a particularly challenging one. It doesn't really matter what your time is the first time you test. What matters most is that you improve your time the next time you're tested.

Congratulations! You've just given yourself a baseline fitness test. As I said, these are not pass/fail tests. They're great fitness markers, and the total-body HIIT workouts in this book should help with any imbalances or weaknesses. (That's one reason I broke out some of the workouts into upper and lower body, core, and so on: so you can give certain areas more work if you want to.) When you rerun the battery 4 weeks from now, I'm betting you'll see an inspiring, even eye-popping transformation. I'm not exaggerating. In this game, it's not whether you win or lose but how much you improve.

These are your first steps. Get ready for more!

## CHAPTER SIX

# MOTIVATION, INSPIRATION, AND HOW TO MAKE HEALTHY CHANGES STICK

I know the secret to motivation.

There's just one problem. *Knowing doesn't matter.* That's the sucker's bet. That's the mirage. Why do I say that? Well, I spend a lot of time trying to motivate people to take care of themselves. In developing my unique blend of fitness and medicine, I've realized that some people need encouragement, others need community, and some need competition. Everyone has something that makes her tick, and over time I've developed strategies to make each person who crosses my path as enthusiastic about taking the medicine of exercise as I am.

My approach is different than the gym's. When my team surveyed some of the thousands of people who have participated in our Ironstrength classes, more than 90 percent said that they view our program differently (in a good way!) from other fitness programs because it's a physician-led workout, and thus they were more likely to participate. So being a doctor helps me motivate folks. I use all the tools unique to the profession to help inspire people to exercise: office visits, free fitness classes, and—if they live somewhere other than the city where I

work—DVDs, e-mail newsletters, online fitness tracker apps, and social media. I also travel a lot for public speaking events about exercise, sports medicine, and how people can keep their bodies running well and injury free. Improving fitness is part of that. So is weight loss. These are big challenges for the average person, so I try to offer some motivation and inspiration along the way in my talks.

So what's the secret to motivation? Well, the big hint is that it has nothing to do with what you know (like I said). But it does have to do with a bunch of other things rattling around in your brain.

### BETWEEN A ROCK AND A GOOD PLACE

I start my lectures with a rock. Literally. I show the audience a rock and I say, "Unless you've been living under one, you know that exercise is good for you."

It's true. I don't think I'm going out on a very thin limb when I say that the vast majority of people know what they need to do to improve their health. The message is ubiquitous—on TV, on newsstands, online—and it goes something like this.

- Eat a balanced diet of lean proteins, good fats, and lots of fruits and vegetables.

- Avoid processed junk foods, saturated and trans fats, and too much sodium.

- Exercise regularly.

- Don't smoke or drink alcohol to excess.

- Sleep well.

Do any of those things surprise you or make you say, "Hmmm, that's really interesting, I never heard that before"? Of course not. We've heard them so often that just about everyone would consider those bits of advice to be common sense. *But knowledge doesn't matter*—if these five principles are so well known and so smart, how come only a small percentage of the population lives by them? The health, wellness, and weight-loss industries are *massive*, which tells me that people know what to do and have an interest in improving themselves, and yet two-thirds of the US population remains overweight or obese. People take weight off and put it back on. People set a goal to run a 5K race, do it, and stop running. People eat healthy for a couple of weeks and then let the old habits regain control.

Why? It's not lack of knowledge or opportunity or resources. People simply have a very hard time staying motivated. There's a disconnect between knowing and doing.

I'm generalizing, of course. The truth is that every single person in the developed world wages a battle of temptation every day—between food choices (the salmon or the deep-fried shrimp), couch choices (to lie about or not to lie about), recreational choices (to have a drink and watch TV or go outside and do something active), and health choices (to schedule an annual physical or not schedule one, thus avoiding any potential bad news). This is the downside of a developed society—all of our conveniences take the effort out of a lot of things.

Now, before we go blaming all those outside influences for the ills of society, let's put the focus back where it needs to be: on you. Are you motivated? Well, you're reading this book, so I have to think you're at least motivated right now, at this moment. Which is awesome—as you'll see in a second, we can work with that. But will you stay motivated? Can you carry through the desire to live healthier, exercise more, and fix bad habits for weeks? Months? Years?

This kind of follow-through comes naturally to some, but to others? Not so much.

## DO YOU "TIRE" EASILY?

So how do you go from living under a rock to working out? Here's an example I use often.

I grew up in Missouri. As you might guess, there's a farm or two in Missouri. Farms have tractors, and those tractors need really big, really heavy tires. If you want to make a big change in your life—exercise regularly or lose weight or eat better—you're staring down the equivalent of a big tractor tire lying on its side in a field. How do you get it—your desired change—up and moving? Well, you gotta spit in your hands, lift hard, muscle that tire upright, and push it until it's moving.

Not easy, right? Exactly.

But what happens when you put in that effort and get that tire up and moving? Rolling the tire is easier than lifting it, right? Starting a new, better, healthier habit is hard. But once you start, keeping it going can be easier, just like rolling a tire. As you roll it along, however, new problems arise. Roads don't all run downhill, and the wind can change. Will you be as interested in rolling that tire uphill? Into a wind? *Ya know what? This kinda stinks. I don't really like my tire anymore.*

Maybe you walk away from the tire. Maybe the tire rolls back down the hill, hits a bump, and flops over on its side again.

Now you're back at square one. If you want to try again, you have to lift that tire up and get it rolling. Meanwhile, if you'd had just a little perspective on motivation, you'd still be rolling that tire and would eventually have gotten it over the hill to a nice, breezy, downhill slope.

So let's talk about the secret to motivation.

## BE TRIGGER HAPPY

Everyone knows a person who has transformed his life—lost a lot of weight or made permanent lifestyle changes or achieved some impressive fitness goal. And not only did he do it, he kept on doing it. And, of course, everyone knows someone (or a lot of someones) who gave it a shot, made it work for a while, but ultimately backslid into the old ways. Maybe that was you?

What's the difference between the successful transformation artist and the wannabe? Is one person superior to the other? No. Is one person stronger, mentally and physically, than the other? Not necessarily. Is one person smarter than the other? IQ doesn't have much to do with it—both folks are intelligent enough to recognize that change would be beneficial. Does one person have more information or resources than the other? Nope, we've already established that the knowledge is out there for everyone to use (or ignore, in many cases).

So what's the big secret?

A person who applies all the knowledge and resources—and does the work necessary—to change her life has decided *I'm doing this; this isn't a quick fix, this is the new me.* And that decision came from a place of serious emotional depth. Something reached this person on a level deep enough to flip a switch, pull a trigger—choose your metaphor. That's the secret. Knowledge is just a tool you can use or ignore. But the motivation to use it—once and for all—comes from that emotionally driven decision.

*I'm doing this; this isn't a quick fix, this is the new me.*

What pulls that emotional trigger? Well, it could be any of the following:

- **You have a health reality check** like a prediabetes diagnosis, a bad blood test, a doctor's stern warning (hey, some folks listen to doctors!), or some other undeniable and ominous health signal.

- **You experience a terrifying health incident**. This is bigger than just a reality check (people can ignore those): chest pains, waking up with blurry vision, nerve pain in your feet. Something that sets off alarms in your body and brain and screams, *This is serious! Listen up!*

- **A terrifying health incident happens to someone you love.** Dad dies of a thunderclap heart attack. Mom's hospitalized because she ignored diabetes symptoms. A sibling receives a cancer diagnosis. Your best friend suddenly has liver problems (time to pay the freight for all those happy hours and lost weekends).

- **Your body fails an unexpected fitness test.** You have to make some sudden movement to avoid danger or sprint to catch a plane or climb stairs to the nosebleed seats at a football game, and you must stop to catch your breath. And you realize that you're more out of shape than you ever dreamed. Embarrassingly so.

- **You see a picture or video of yourself** and wonder, *How did that happen?*

- **Your kids deliver the revelation.** Maybe you can't run around with them anymore, or they make an innocent comment in public about your body or all the cookies you like to eat. Or maybe you just realize, like a lot of parents, that if you stay on the road you're on, your life with them might not be as long as you once thought.

- **You're happy on the outside but truly sad on the inside** about your physical condition and lifestyle. And you're sick of sad. You've had sad up to here.

That's just a sampling. In theory, it could be anything—people's triggers are as unique as their DNA. But something happens that touches them at the deepest level, and they have what alcoholics call a moment of clarity. And it shakes them. Others have described it as finding your "why," or your true reason for doing something.

And just like that: change.

## CAN YOU PULL YOUR OWN TRIGGER?

Looking at that list, you might think that this big trigger-pulling moment is something you have to wait for or stumble upon, like an addict having to hit rock bottom before asking for help. That's crazy. That kind of thinking goes back to the knowledge phenomenon, about knowing something and not acting upon it. If you know that eating better and exercising more are the paths to better health and you don't do them, then you have other bits of knowledge you're not acting upon, either: You know you're overweight or sedentary or trapped in an addictive habit like smoking or drinking too much. Maybe it's even simpler: You're relatively healthy and relatively active, but you know you're leaving so much potential on the table.

Heck yes, you can pull your own trigger. Why wait?

Starting is simple: Review your life and think of times when your lifestyle or bad habit may have triggered a reaction in you. Maybe no one ever knew. Maybe it was just something you saw or experienced. And maybe you felt a finger on your trigger—pressure but not a pull. Analyze that moment, review that emotion, find out what about it resonated with you so much. Now all you have to do is embrace it.

Finding your trigger point may also be as simple as thinking about what's important to you: family, friends, or even the only-you things that have meaning, like wanting to

# Follow the Money, Find Your Truth

Here's a little motivational self-test that might open your eyes. Now, when it comes to habits—good and bad—a lot of people are happy to let you know how they roll. "I live a really healthy lifestyle" or "I'm going to run that half-marathon" or "I only have a couple drinks on the weekend." Maybe they do. And hey, maybe *you* do. But if you want to know where your real priorities lie, if what you tell yourself and others is true, what is deep-down important to you above all else, then put your claims to the test.

Look at your bank account and credit card statements.

That's right. How you spend money reveals your true priorities across all areas of your life. You'll see how you picked up some extra alcohol at the liquor store. Or had a night out eating wings at the pub. Or drank 500-calorie lattes at the coffee bar four times last week.

You'll also see how often you had lunch at the health food restaurant. Or bought a case of sports drinks at the grocery store. Or yet another pair of workout shoes. You'll see how much you spent at the gym or traveling for athletic events or at the produce market.

Numbers don't lie. But sometimes we lie to ourselves.

Maybe you don't know just how much you spend on that little something now and then. Maybe you just don't think about it. Or maybe your habits are already pretty great. In any case, it's a worthwhile test, especially if you want to commit to living a healthier life.

achieve a big athletic goal or write a book or start a nonprofit. Big things. The kind of things that, left undone, will make you feel regret—a seriously deep emotion if there ever was one—and help you see that all that knowledge is just noise in your head unless you finally take action.

Now here's the interesting part: Once you think about something that means a lot to you, measure it against all the things that have held you back—bad habits, distractions, laziness, procrastination, the comfort of the couch or the lure of the junk food/booze/late nights—and decide what's more important to you. Because if you think about it, up until now all those negative things have held more sway in your head than the positive. Oh, yes, they have. You've prioritized the bad and put the good on the back burner. Which one do you truly want?

Now . . . make your choice.
Pull your trigger.

## THE LONG VIEW

I've talked a lot about tires and triggers, emotions and motivation, and that's fine. But let's say you pull that trigger and decide to commit to something very simple: regular workouts from this book. (That's why we're here, right?) You try a few workouts and enjoy them. You make them part of your routine—it's easy to do, and you've been using the 10-minute, 20-minute, and full 30-minute options to make it happen. All is well.

Then one day you have to sacrifice a workout because life gets in the way: a work project or some unexpected and unavoidable time-suck. "I'll go back at it tomorrow," you say. Maybe you do. And maybe you don't. Maybe the work project kept you up late and you opt to sleep in rather than roll out of bed for the workout.

Recognize the pattern? Exactly. Day to day, it can be difficult to maintain the motivation necessary to make your workout a priority, a habit, something you really don't want to skip.

Starting out? It can be exciting, interesting, a novelty that feels really good because you know you've made that good change and you're seeing gains. But excitement can wane; interest, flag; and novelty, wear off. I'm about as big an exercise fanatic as you'll ever meet. I almost never skip a day because I love how exercise feels and how it sets me up for better performance in everything I do—I'm energized, engaged, and able to work at a higher level for a longer period. But do I have days where other commitments attack my exercise time? Or days when I'm just not feeling it? Sure I do. Here's how I handle them.

- **Forgive and fight another day.** If skipping the workout is unavoidable, well, it happens. Cut yourself some slack and get back to it tomorrow. You may feel frustrated or even angry at whatever forces have conspired to mess up your routine, but trust me, the negativity isn't worth it. Think about how good the movement will feel the next day. This is my primary strategy, and I'm always feeling good about it afterward.

- **Sneak in movement (aka be NEAT).** It's not a workout, but spare moments happen all day long, and you can fill them with movement. Become a stealth squatter. Stand or pace if you don't have to sit. This keeps your workout top of mind even when you don't have time for it. Multiple studies have shown that building in fitness during the day, increasing your NEAT (non-exercise activity thermogenesis) profile, leads to dramatic health benefits. What is NEAT? The energy you burn in any activity other than eating, sleeping, and exercising—in other words, all the other stuff you do in a given day. These can be easy things like taking the stairs, walking or biking to work, or even playing with the dog. While at work, a standing desk might make a difference, or try a walking break during the day. The American Heart Association and American College of Sports Medicine both support 10,000 steps per day, about 3 miles of walking, to meet the daily requirement for movement. Everything adds up—even fidgeting at your desk counts. Increasingly, companies are incentivizing employees to build fitness into their daily lives. They aren't doing this because they're good Samaritans. Rather, they realize that employees who move are healthier, take fewer sick days, and are more cost effective. When you're thinking about your day, think: *I'm mobile, I'm flexible, I'm dynamic.* Those aren't bad thoughts to have in the middle of a long workday.

- **Start anyway and see what happens.** This one is my favorite. I have the 10-minute workout option in this book for a reason. Time is precious. A 10-minute-or-less workout isn't ideal, but if you hit it hard, it can be a difference maker. Even if it's been the worst day ever and you have no time and you have no motivation, just start exercising. Maybe you'll have to cut it short. But maybe after a couple of minutes, you'll start to feel better. Maybe you'll get into it more and more as you go. Maybe your lousy mood will brighten. And maybe, just maybe, you'll squeeze in more time than you thought or work harder and fit more into the time you have. Or maybe, best of all, once you're into it, you won't stop until *you* decide you're done. It's so simple: Start moving, because once you start, you might just keep going.

## MAKE THIS THING *YOUR* THING

Here's one last motivational secret: Make your workouts irresistible. Sound like a pipe dream? Not really. And if you can do it, you're golden. You won't miss. You won't just do your workouts, you'll savor them. Imagine savoring a workout. Imagine feeling sad not because you have to start but because you have to stop.

I've been in that sweet spot for years. You can get there, too. How? Just make exercise your Thing. Everyone has his or her Thing. Exercise and sports medicine are my Things. When something is your Thing, it's not about dedication. It's just what you do. And that can be so strong that even the word *motivation* is no longer necessary. Almost sounds crazy, right? You're so motivated that motivation isn't part of the process. That's the sweet spot, right there.

So how does something become your

Thing? In my experience, between what I see from my patients and people in my fitness classes and others I meet in my travels, it varies. Some folks prefer full immersion. They just dive in. That can work wonders, but it can also make you realize that no, this activity is not your Thing, nor will it ever be. Some people build gradually. Some hate an activity to start with but grow into it so passionately and deeply that you'd never know it wasn't their Thing.

In a way it's a bit like falling in love. You can't predict how it will happen, you just know when it's working. Could be love at first sight. Could be a slow burn. Could be repulsion at first sight, too, but coupled with a strange magnetism that brings you back and pulls you in permanently. I don't think we need to make this a Mystery of Life, however (he said with a grin). Let's just talk about ways you can make your Thing happen. Consider some of these ideas:

- **Appreciate this Thing (which is not yet *your* Thing) as a positive force in your life.** I capitalize the word *Thing* throughout this chapter deliberately because if you do that in your own brain, you'll think of exercise as something significant. That's a good place to start. *This is a positive force in my life and I feel great about it.* The goal here is to revel in the positivity. The goal is getting to where you look forward to it. And when it finally becomes your Thing? You'll feel possessive and want to protect it.

- **Keep your Thing front and center—and simple.** To me, there's nothing more powerful than a pair of sneakers. They're your companions on the exercise journey. They're your buddies, keeping your feet comfortable and cushioned and moving you forward. I don't go so far as naming my running shoes, but I don't discourage the practice in others (I'm winking here, okay?). So here's my tip: Give your sneaks—or whatever exercise gear feels like a talisman to you—a place of honor in your home; ideally, somewhere that will keep them in your field of vision and, thus, keep exercise top of mind. Maybe it's right by the front door. Maybe it's by your bed. Maybe it's over the fireplace. Wherever it is, make it prominent enough that when company comes over, you can point to the shoes (or whatever your talisman is) and say, "Those are my new friends. Would you like to meet my new friends? Just don't touch them. Only I can touch them." (Okay, this is silly, but my point is that you can have a lot of fun with this.) When exercise is on your brain in a serious but fun way, it remains always a positive and joyful Thing, not something you've been sentenced to.

- **Play small ball—at first.** Small steps, small goals, small victories—every gain is golden when you're starting out. What should not be small? Your celebrations, rewards, and smiles. And as you accumulate all those small things? Steps, goals, and victories will grow larger. You'll want them. And the workouts you're doing will prepare you. Look forward to success!

- **Bring friends.** You've no doubt heard that exercising with a buddy can make the process more enjoyable and harder to skip. All true. But thinking bigger is a theme in this book, so let's do just that. An exercise buddy is good, but an exercise *army* is great. One of the things I'm most proud of is the network of active people—literally thousands—that I've been able to assemble through my practice, my Ironstrength fitness classes, and the sheer magnetism of exercise itself. The Internet, e-mail, and social media keep all of us connected and—here's the most important part—involved. Man, when you feel involved in something, a genuine part of a force for good, it's incredible. Like you can do anything. So don't just find an exercise buddy. Join clubs, be active, meet new people, and work toward assembling an exercise army. You won't want to skip a workout. Ever.

- **Sprint downhill.** I don't mean literally—you could face-plant. What I mean is, when you're feeling good about exercise and how well you're doing with it, when the sun is out and you're fully motivated, when you wake up and know it's going to be a good day—*that's when you push harder.* When you run downhill or with the wind or whenever forces are working with you instead of against you, the instinct is to enjoy it and take it easy. Nope. Go harder. Take advantage of the good feelings. Life doesn't always give you a nice tailwind. This is the time to set a new goal or try to push to a new level. This is also the time to celebrate your Thing and how great it makes you feel.

Buy a new pair of friends, er, shoes. Get some of your army together. Revel in your Thing. You've earned every one of those good feelings.

## KEEP THAT TIRE ROLLING

By now you're getting it: Putting forth an honest effort and surrounding yourself with positive influences are the two biggest keys to long-term life changes. People (myself included) can invent catchy new ways of offering advice and support, bring a fresh perspective, and pull for you as hard as they can, but in the end it's always going to come down to those two things. They'll keep your tire rolling. And no matter what, the end result will always be up to you!

## CHAPTER SEVEN

# REST, RECOVER, REJUVENATE

I do love my exercise. When I'm working out, I'm happy. It's that simple. But I also know that some of the most important health and fitness magic happens *between* workouts. In a nutshell, your off hours can make your next workout better or worse—and also affect your long-term health and fitness. How is that possible? It's all about your approach to rest, recovery, and rejuvenation.

People have different philosophies about rest. For some, just sticking to a set regimen is enough: "I exercise three times a week, that's it; I'm happy with that." Those folks don't do any other activities on their off days and don't take any special approach to recovery. Work out, live life. You know what? That's okay. But if that's your MO, you should know that you're leaving some potential on the table. (And please don't take that as a criticism; I know it's a battle for most people to carve out time for exercise, and doing it three times a week consistently is a major win all by itself.)

But if exercise is your Thing (see the previous chapter) or you want it to be, how you handle rest, recovery, and rejuvenation is part of the package. This falls under the umbrella of "thinking bigger" when it comes to fitness.

As you've read previously, I recommend exercising 7 days a week. That does not mean you should be doing the HIIT workouts in this book 7 days a week or even 4 days a week. But I recommend some kind of physical activity every day, even if you consider it a "rest day." I think of it this way: If your workouts are all about breaking your body down, all those other hours should build it back up.

Let's talk about that downtime, shall we?

## WHAT IS REST?

A nice word, isn't it? It evokes pleasant images: chilling next to a pool, lying in a hammock, or sleeping in on a Sunday. Maybe rest means a getaway to you. Maybe it simply means the opposite of *work*. All of that sounds great. But for the purposes of this book—and revamping your workout philosophy—I think we need to revamp our definition of *rest*.

Let's put it this way: Rest is a conscious, deliberate approach to how you use the time between workouts. Rest is therapeutic. Rest is restorative. And—this is the most important part—rest is dynamic.

Dynamic rest? You bet. To me, dynamic rest (some folks refer to it as active rest) is the best kind. What do I mean by "dynamic rest"? Light to moderate activities that get you moving—and even perspiring—but don't work your body like your exercise regimen does. The key is to avoid overuse and allow your body to recover from the "real" workouts. For example, if you're all about the strength HIIT in this book, go for a bike ride or take a yoga class on an off day (more on yoga later). If you jog, lift some weights. Do something light. Do something for fun. Throw a Frisbee or football. Play a round of golf. Find a pool. Or maybe just get out for a brisk walk with your dog or some friends.

In a way, dynamic rest is something that allows you to feel relaxed. What regular exercise takes out, dynamic rest should put back in. These activities engage your brain, allowing you to reflect and enjoy being active and what your body can do. Also, doing things that engage your brain as well as your hands and eyes can become meditative: gardening, crafts, even hauling and folding laundry (the only thing that makes it a chore is your approach to it!). The point is to keep moving and engage your body whenever you can.

# Is There Ever a Time for Total Rest?

In general, I'm not a fan of lying around (those who know me best would consider this an understatement!). However, there are times when your body tells you to dial it back and take a break. The problem is that this is a feeling—totally subjective, with no gauge or number or test to consult—and if you've had issues sticking to a dedicated exercise regimen in the past, giving yourself "a break" may not be what you need. Everyone gets sore after a good workout. And you're not exactly an outlier if you feel stiff getting out of bed the day after, either. If you truly need a day of total rest, give yourself the gift. But think of it that way—as a gift or special occasion. One way to decide if you're worthy of this gift? Ask yourself the following questions.

1. *Am I injured?* This is different than being sore. You'll feel pain in the affected area. If so, I still don't recommend total rest. (See Part Three for a lot more detail on this.)

2. *Did I get enough sleep?* A full night's rest does wonders for your mental and physical outlook, even if you worked yourself hard the previous day (more on sleep in just a moment). Lousy rest makes you feel lousy. My suggestion: Move! Dynamic rest will wake you up.

3. *Am I really sore or tired, or am I just not feeling it today?* Be honest. There's nothing wrong with a mental health day. But there's a difference between that and avoiding exercise.

4. *What's my fitness level?* This isn't a trick question. Sure, the answer requires subjectivity, but if you're a beginner to these HIIT workouts or someone relatively fit who just started adding in strength HIIT, giving your body some time to adapt isn't a bad idea. Still, I suggest some dynamic rest— even gentle dynamic rest—as opposed to any extended time on the couch.

Ultimately, you're the decision maker on total rest. Just be honest with yourself about what you truly need.

Steps and reps add up, and that's how you build up to living an active lifestyle. After a while, it's the only life you'll want.

Now let's talk about other ways to be kind to your body.

## THE MOST IMPORTANT ACTIVITY OF YOUR DAY

Do you know what it is? I'll give you a hint: It's not your workout; neither is it your job nor the time you spend with family and friends. In fact, it's nothing you do during any waking moment of your day.

Which leaves only one thing: your non-waking moments. Yes, I'm talking about sleep. And I'm not kidding: It truly is the most important activity of your day.

Why? Sleep is a necessary time of regeneration—in fact, while drifting off and floating in your personal dream world feels easy and warm and relaxing, the hours ahead are, in their way, a very intense time for your body. Some amazing work happens while you're dozing. Muscle rebuilds itself, bone strengthens, red blood cells restock. Not to mention how important REM sleep is to restoring your brain and keeping the physical organ—as well as the psychological functions it manages—in top condition. But keeping with the theme of exercise: High-quality sleep is the true rest that transforms all the effort you exert into a stronger, healthier, and more energized body.

Now, with all that said, can you say that you get the 7 to 8 hours of high-quality sleep that you need every night?

Didn't think so. Few people do. The average person gets 6.8 hours per night, according to poll information from Gallup. Sixty-five percent of people get 7 hours or less, and 40 percent get less than 6 hours. For perspective, back in the pre-TV-Internet-smartphone culture of 1942, 45 percent got 8 hours a

## What's Messing with Your Sleep?

When you consider all the things that can disrupt your slumber, it's amazing that the average person can function at all during the day. Which ones affect you?

| | | |
|---|---|---|
| Obesity | Work schedule | Racing thoughts |
| Sleep apnea | Snoring | Caffeine |
| Parenthood | Bedmate's snoring | Alcohol |
| Too much phone time | Outside noise | Nicotine |
| Too much tablet time | TV noise | Recreational drugs |
| Too much computer time | Stress | Prescription drugs |
| Pets | Illness | Uncomfortable room temperature |
| Seasonal allergies | Hormonal changes (from PMS to menopause) | Bad dreams |
| Insomnia | | |

night and only 11 percent got less than 6 hours. And there was a world war on!

Of all the factors that shortchange our sleep, the one that's probably ignored the most is deliberate choice. Sleep is the first thing to take a hit in the name of lifestyle and career, whether because we're pushing ourselves to work more hours or sacrificing sleep so we can fit in more life. Maybe you don't feel like you have a choice. Young children, intense jobs, and long commutes don't exactly make a person feel like she has options. We always think we can "get by" on less sleep.

Well, there are consequences. Lack of sleep is linked to higher blood pressure, weight gain, elevated stress hormones, and other things that will detract not just from your athletic performance but also your general health.

I'm a doctor, so I have to say it: You need to prioritize sleep. It may not be easy, but think of it like this: You're learning to prioritize exercise, so do the same for sleep. Make it a package deal. One is your daylight priority; the other, your nighttime priority. You may have heard these common-sense sleep helpers before, but they work, so they bear repeating.

- Make bedtime a routine: same time, same wind-down ritual.

- Lay off the following things at least 2 hours before bed: electronic screens, food, and booze. And, horrible as it sounds, don't have any caffeine after 3 p.m.

- Transform your bedroom into a snoozing paradise as best you can: Keep it dark, quiet, and cool.

- Hit your mental reset button and enjoy the drift into slumber. It feels really good!

And if all else fails? Sleep in on weekends if you can, and don't underestimate the power of the catnap. Napping for 20 minutes or less in the middle of the day can be transformative.

Now, let's talk about some things that might help you sleep better.

## MUCH-NEEDED KNEADING

A lot of people equate massage with spas and indulgent special occasions. But I'd like you to think of massage as essential total-body therapy that's for more than just sore muscles. Regular massage has so many benefits.

- Moderate-pressure massage activates the parasympathetic nervous system, which controls involuntary activities like heart rate and digestion, and may help lower blood pressure. Meanwhile, it may increase white blood cell count and decrease stress hormones like cortisol and vasopressin. The potential result: better immune function.

- Studies show that massage leads to favorable results for a whole list of medical problems, including lower-back pain, knee arthritis, headaches, constipation, carpal tunnel syndrome, restless legs syndrome, and stroke. Massage may even provide pain relief in cancer patients.

- Massage enhances mobility and flexibility.

- It could also help you sleep better. I remember something about sleep being important . . . now, where did I read that?

Here are some popular types of massage—readily available just about anywhere—and what sets them apart from one another (this is by no means a complete list).

- **Swedish massage.** This is the classic rubdown, with soothing, flowing strokes and, sometimes, percussion (tapping or pounding), all of which are designed to boost circulation. Some therapists like to use hot stones, as well.

- **Shiatsu massage.** In Japanese, *shiatsu* translates as "finger pressure," though the actual technique involves targeted massage of points along the body's meridians, which are the tracks through which chi, or energy, is thought to flow. (Western medical practitioners aren't fully convinced that chi exists, but some theorize that it's energy flowing along nerve pathways.)

- **Myofascial release.** Muscles are covered in a connective tissue called fascia that can become very tight, to the point of causing pain. Relieving that tension loosens muscles and improves your mobility. This is a deeper massage.

- **Trigger point massage.** When muscles tighten, they can squeeze nerves and cause pain that radiates to other areas. This massage style delivers deep pressing on specific points around the body that can cause pain in wider areas, maintaining pressure on a trigger point until it "releases."

- **Thai massage.** Sometimes called Thai yoga massage, this technique involves massage

and assisted stretching to help muscles relax and loosen, while improving circulation to reduce any soreness.

## DIY Massage (for Cheap!)

Sixty minutes with a massage pro is a wonderful thing. And expensive! But you can give your muscles regular self-massage with some simple tools. A tennis ball is great for rolling the bottoms of your feet (and preventing plantar fasciitis), and it just plain feels good. A massage stick (aka muscle roller) is small enough to keep in a desk drawer and provides the perfect 5-minute break, especially if you spend much of the day sitting.

For the best do-it-yourself results, however, nothing beats a foam roller. One of the best favors you can do for your body is some foam rolling every night in front of the TV (you can do it anytime, anywhere, of course, but in front of the TV is *so-o-o* convenient). Just run through the following basic rolling routine—after a couple of times, you'll have it memorized—and you'll be done before the first commercial break.

A few quick notes about foam rolling:

- Just 30 to 60 seconds on a muscle should do the trick.

- Roll muscle, not bone (so stop, for example, before the roller hits your knee).

- On some areas, you might feel discomfort as you roll. That's normal and, in a way, a really good sign. It's proof that the area is tight and needs the work. Regular rolling will reduce or eliminate the pain over time as your muscles loosen up.

### GLUTES FOAM ROLL

Sit on a foam roller, with it positioned under your right glute. Cross your right leg over the top of your left thigh. Put your hands on the floor for support. Roll your body forward and backward in small movements so the roller massages your lower glute to your upper glute. Repeat with the roller under your left glute.

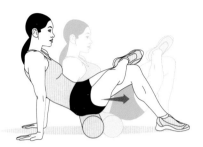

### ILIOTIBIAL BAND (IT BAND) FOAM ROLL

Lie on your right side and place your right hip on a foam roller. Put your hands on the floor for support. Cross your left leg over your right, and place your left foot flat on the floor. Roll your body forward and backward in small movements until the roller reaches just above your knee. Repeat on the other side.

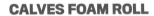

### CALVES FOAM ROLL

Sit on the floor and stretch your legs out in front of your body. Place a foam roller under your right calf with your right leg straight. Cross your left ankle over your right ankle. Put your hands flat on the floor for support, and raise your body off the floor while keeping your back naturally arched. Roll your body forward until the roller has crossed your entire calf region. Roll back and forth. Repeat with the roller under your left calf.

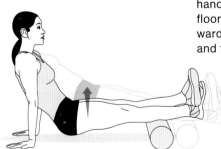

## QUADS FOAM ROLL

Lie facedown on the floor with a foam roller positioned above both of your knees. Using your hands and lower arms to stabilize yourself, slowly roll your body over the roller until it reaches the tops of your thighs. Roll back and forth.

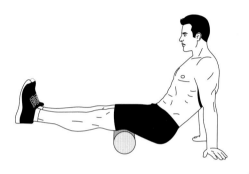

## HAMSTRINGS FOAM ROLL

Sit on a foam roller with it positioned just below your left glute, at the top of your left hamstring. Put your hands on the floor for support. Roll your body forward and back-ward along the length of your hamstring. Repeat with the roller under your right hamstring. (For a wide roller, you can do both hamstrings at once.)

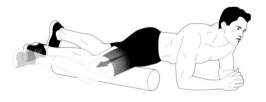

## GROIN FOAM ROLL

Lie facedown on the floor. Place a foam roller parallel to your body. Raise up on your elbows for support. Position your right thigh nearly perpendicular to your body, with the inner portion of your thigh just above the level of your knee, resting on top of the roller. Roll your body toward the right until the roller reaches your pelvis. Then roll back and forth. Repeat on your left thigh.

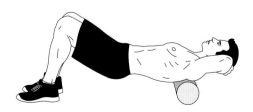

## THORACIC SPINE FOAM ROLL

Lie faceup with a foam roller under your upper back, at the tops of your shoulder blades. Cross your arms over your chest or clasp them behind your head. Your knees should be bent, with your feet flat on the floor. Raise your hips so they're slightly elevated off the floor. Roll back and forth over your shoulder blades and your mid-back and upper back.

## EVERYDAY YOGA

Yoga is everywhere, you hear about it all the time, and yet I still think it's underrated. It's the perfect dynamic rest activity for days you're not doing HIIT. Just one basic yoga class a week can help build athleticism and flexibility. Try this brief routine after a workout or as a way of de-stressing and focusing your energy during the day.

For best results, hold each *asana*, or pose, for 30 seconds to 1 minute, breathing deeply and slowly through your nose. Breathing is key. If you are unable to perform the pose as described without undue discomfort, back off a bit (reaching for your shins rather than feet on the Forward Bend or placing a small block or bench underneath your hands, for example). As with anything, the more you do yoga, the better you'll get.

Although asanas appear to be static, they are actually very active: As you breathe, you will probably find yourself able to deepen into each stretch.

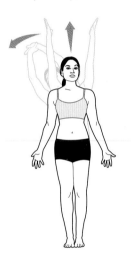

### MOUNTAIN

Stand with your feet together and big toes touching. Relax your shoulders and lengthen your neck. Let your arms relax along your sides, palms to the front, and gaze forward. Optional: Raise your arms straight above your head, palms facing in, elbows facing out. Add in a side stretch by leaning to one side, then repeating for the other side.

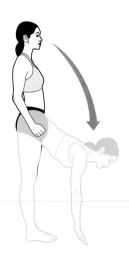

### FORWARD BEND

Stand with your feet together, arms at your side. Exhale as you bend forward at your hips, reaching your hands toward the floor. Imagine folding your body in half. (Note: For beginners, bend as far as you can and hold for 30 seconds, making sure to breathe slowly and deeply.)

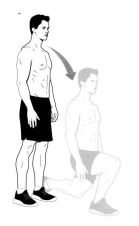

## DEEP LUNGE

Stand with your feet shoulder-width apart. Step forward with your right leg and lower yourself until your right leg is bent 90 degrees and your left knee is almost touching the floor. Keep your weight resting on the heel of your front foot and the ball of your rear foot. Raise your arms straight up over your head, keeping them shoulder-width apart. Keeping your arms straight, bring your palms together. Hold for 30 seconds, return to the starting position, and repeat for the left leg.

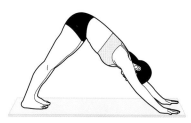

## DOWNWARD-FACING DOG

Begin on all fours with your knees hip-width apart and your hands shoulder-width apart. Your hips should be over your knees and your shoulders over your wrists. Walk your hands a few inches in front of your shoulders. Curl your toes under, lift your hips, and straighten your legs. Push into your palms to draw more energy into your lower body to help elevate your pelvis. Keep your arms straight and so that your body forms an upside-down V.

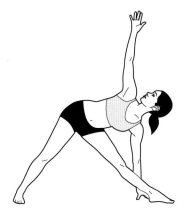

## TRIANGLE

Stand with your feet one leg-length apart. Rotate your left foot out to a 90-degree angle and your right foot inward to a 45-degree angle, keeping your heels aligned. Lift your arms out to your sides until they're parallel to the floor. Bend to your left and extend your left arm to the floor outside your left ankle. Your right arm should point to the sky, and your right shoulder should align vertically with your left. Keep your core engaged and your legs straight. Hold for the specified time, then do the opposite side.

# PART THREE

# Pains, Strains, and... Gains?

The workouts in this book will keep you moving, but this section will help when your body tells you to stop. See, sometimes doing what's good for you—living an active life—can hurt. Our bodies are a collection of interconnected moving parts, and parts can break down. I see dozens of patients each week, bringing a variety of complaints, yet all are bound by one truth: They want to heal so they can get moving again. Here we'll take a look at 22 of the most common sports injuries and how to approach them so you can keep exercising and still achieve your fitness gains—so much so that by the time you feel 100 percent, you might actually be at 110.

## CHAPTER EIGHT

# "OUCH" HAPPENS

Every day, I see the ecstasy and agony of exercise, the warriors and the wounded. I meet people who simply love movement, that they can run and jump or join in my Iron-strength classes in New York City or cross the finish line of a race they trained for weeks to conquer. Then there's the other side: people I treat who can't move how they'd like to because they're injured.

"Ouch!" happens. In fact, if you're an active person, I'd say that ouch—in some form—is inevitable. Even the most perfectly trained body can break down. It can happen in so many ways: pushing yourself too hard, overuse, putting just enough stress on a muscle or ligament that's not ready for it, or plain old bad luck. Just like that, your ecstasy turns into agony.

In this special section, I'll show you what to do for 22 of the most common sports injuries—from the bottom of your feet (plantar fasciitis) all the way up to your neck. Most injuries respond very well to home-based care, so I offer a host of tips and treatments for each. Some cases go beyond just the ouch, however, and could be serious. I'll let you know when you should call a doctor.

Before we dig in, though, I want to talk about something important: your smile.

"My what?" you ask.

Just stay with me.

Injured people have one thing in common—besides feeling some level of pain—and I see it in every patient I treat: They've lost their smiles. Healthy, active people smile all the time—they have freedom of movement, and it feels great. But take that freedom away? It sucks the life right out of you. I felt it myself when I blew out my knee in medical school. It's more than just a disruption of your physical life—it's a blow to your psyche. Whether the injury is a minor annoyance or a major rehab project, your entire psychology changes, and not in a good way.

I try to offer advice, ideas, and motivation to people no matter which side of the equation they may be on, whether I meet them in a fitness class or in my exam room. And because of that, I know one thing to be true—and it may be the most important piece of advice I can offer.

If you get hurt, *keep moving*.

Now, I don't mean that if you pull a hamstring, you should keep running. Or that if you think you tore your ACL playing basketball, you should finish out the game. (I'm fanatical about exercise but not crazy!) What I do mean: An injury is not a vacation from exercise. So much so that as a doctor, I believe that suggesting "total rest" after an injury is not just bad advice, but bad medicine. You can certainly rest the body part that needs to heal, but *keep moving*. There are smart ways you can exercise without aggravating your injury, but you have to remain committed to staying active even though the ouch has taken some wind out of your sails. Don't think of it as "playing through the pain," which isn't very smart. Think of it as playing around the pain.

Why do this, besides the fact that exercise is so good for you? Well, let's break down what happens after the typical sports injury.

## *Don't "play through the pain." Play around the pain.*

My knee blowout kept me inactive for months. And it stank. I was miserable. It was not just the day-to-day lack of exercise but also the bigger question of just what my knee would allow me to do long term. What kind of athlete could I be when I was 30, 40, 50 years old? (If I'd only known then what I know now!) I always refer to exercise as a miracle drug, and one of the reasons is the secretion of happy neurotransmitters like serotonin and dopamine during activity. Take that daily dose away and it's easy for the dark clouds to roll in. That's what happened

to me. And it goes beyond a chemical reaction in your brain. Think about what happens when you're unable to do the things you love to do.

- **You get bored.** You focus on the negatives. Exercise is referred to as nature's antidepressant for a reason. The positive mind-body connection that happens during exercise is undeniable. More time on your hands isn't always a good thing.

- **You feel lousy.** Not only does some body part hurt, but you're also not getting your regular dose of feel-good neurotransmitters. Bottom line, you just don't feel as good as you normally do.

- **You lose gains.** Whatever physical shape you've worked hard to achieve will soften. You'll grow weaker, and your cardiovascular health will suffer. And it will take that much more work to get back what you've lost once you're able to train at full speed again. How does that sound? Exactly.

- **You get depressed.** It happened to me. It can happen to you.

## MOVEMENT, MOVEMENT, MOVEMENT

How do you avoid all those negatives? *Keep moving.* Exercise doesn't just make you feel good—it keeps you from feeling bad. Even if your activity is limited, that's better than nothing. You'll keep some of your conditioning. You'll get your dose of the exercise miracle drug. You'll feel better, be more positive, and keep smiling in spite of that little ding. Setback? Move forward. An injury isn't the end of the world or even the end of your workout regimen if you approach fitness with patience and smarts.

How do you do that? Use what I call dynamic rest.

First, rest and rehab your injury. Lay off that body part and do what's required to get it back to full strength. That could mean some home-based remedies you'll find in Chapter 9 or seeing a doctor and using other prescribed interventions. Take your injury seriously and approach it as a problem to be solved, and this book and/or your physician will give you the tools to do it.

Second, *dynamic* means "in motion," so *keep moving* while the rest and rehab go on. Use the following strategies.

**Do something that doesn't aggravate the injury.** If you sprain your ankle, focus on upper-body and core work for a couple of weeks. If you hurt your shoulder, hit your lower body and core. Strain an oblique muscle? No reason not to work everything from the glutes on down until your condition improves.

And guess what? This book has all those possibilities covered for you. Not only does Chapter 9 cover the most common sports injuries and how to treat them, the 30-minute workout section includes a variety of training sessions for your upper body, lower body, and core to go along with all the total-body workouts. Use 'em!

**Hit it hard.** Or should I say "HIIT it hard"? Whatever your limited activity may be, push yourself. You want to feel the burn. You want your heart pounding and lungs heaving. You want to proceed as if the next level is inevitable. Because here's a crazy notion: You could even improve your cardiovascular health—as well as whichever body zone you're working—during your injury rehab. Imagine being fitter after you heal. Imagine how much faster you'll get back to where you were pre-ouch and how much easier you'll push beyond that.

I say it often: If you *keep moving*, you'll be the happiest hurt person on earth.

## CHAPTER NINE

# IDENTIFY AND FIX WHAT'S AILING YOU

## A (Mostly) Complete Catalog of Maladies

# Plantar Fasciitis

### The Symptoms

Nasty pain in the bottom of the foot, especially when running or even taking your first steps out of bed in the morning.

### What's Going On in There?

Plantar fasciitis is inflammation of the plantar fascia. (*Plantar* refers to the bottom of the foot, and *fascia*, in this case, to the band of connective tissue running from your heel bone to the front of the foot.) This tissue helps support your foot's arch, gives it shape, and aids in stability when your foot strikes the ground and then pushes off.

The injury to the fascia usually begins where the fascia connects to the bony bump on the bottom of the heel (called the calcaneal tuberosity, one of the most fun anatomical terms). The inflammation and pain come from excessive tension. The muscles above and the shape of the foot below contribute. The calf muscles (specifically, the gastrocnemius and soleus) connect to the heel bone via the Achilles tendon. When those muscles are tight, the tendon pulls on the bone from above, which stretches the fascia and causes strain. People with high arches are especially prone to plantar fasciitis because the arch itself also contributes tension to the fascia.

A mild case can turn major very quickly. Inflammation makes the fascia more prone to microtears, which can lead to debilitating pain. In other words, you can't walk, let alone exercise.

Bad cases can last months. My youngest brother was once sidelined for 10 months by plantar fasciitis, and I see many patients with similar stories.

### Fix It

- **Employ dynamic rest.** Take a break from the offending activity. The earlier you address plantar fasciitis, the better. How long you need to rest depends on the severity of the case, but expect to be sidelined for at least a couple weeks or more. Stick with intense upper-body activity that

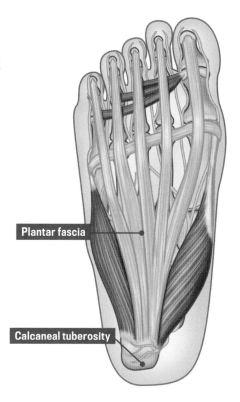

Plantar fascia

Calcaneal tuberosity

doesn't load your foot. Does that stink? Sure. But it beats crippling yourself!

■ **Stretch.** Use the stretches described in Prevent It. Be gentle. Go slow. You're trying to bring relief to the tightness in the area, not prepare for a game or race. As the injury heals, adopt the stretching habit permanently.

■ **Try an NSAID.** An anti-inflammatory like ibuprofen or naproxen can help reduce pain and inflammation.

■ **Ease yourself back into the game.** Don't start strenuous activity until you're pain free. If you mess around with this, you'll simply aggravate the injury and be out even longer.

## Prevent It

■ **Stay flexible.** The best way to stretch this area is to put your toes and the ball of your foot against the top of the vertical edge of a step with your heel on the floor and slowly lean forward, keeping your leg straight, feeling the stretch farther down the leg near the Achilles tendon. Repeat the stretch with your knee bent, feeling the stretch in the lower leg. Hold each stretch for 15 to 20 seconds, and repeat several times in each position. Ideally, you'll do this daily, before and after exercise.

■ **Roll it.** This is a simple preventive measure you can do anywhere, even sitting at your desk at work. Roll a tennis ball back and forth under each foot for a few minutes a day. The movement of the ball massages and loosens the fascia.

■ **Try orthotics.** Over-the-counter rigid arch supports can be helpful, especially for you high-arched folks. Prescription orthotics are another option because they're custom-fitted to your foot, but I suggest (much cheaper) OTC orthotics first—in my practice, about 90 percent of patients have good results with them. If they don't work, then see a podiatrist for a custom set.

## When to Call a Doctor

If symptoms don't improve in about 2 weeks, make an appointment.

The doctor will probably have you do the home remedies listed here, as well as more aggressive treatments, depending on the severity of the condition. These include wearing foot splints at night, keeping sandals with a big arch next to the bed for those first steps in the morning (which can reaggravate the injury before it heals completely), doing physical therapy, or getting corticosteroid injections to ease inflammation.

Another potential therapy is platelet-rich plasma (PRP). In areas of the body that don't have great blood supply, healing is slow. The doctor injects your own platelet-rich plasma back into your body in the injured areas to promote faster healing. The upside is that it works for most people. The downside is that it may not be covered by insurance and is expensive. But if you can't get results from any other therapy, it doesn't hurt to investigate it.

## Do You Need Surgery?

Not likely. Surgery is required only in extreme cases that don't respond to normal treatment.

# Ankle Sprain

## The Symptoms

- **Common ankle sprain:** Results from "rolling" or "twisting" your ankle. Mild sprains (grade 1) cause tolerable pain, some swelling, and some difficulty walking. Severe sprains (grade 3) bring on incredible pain, possible ligament rupture, swelling, bruising, and total joint instability.

- **High ankle sprain:** Usually occurs when foot is inverted and twisted. It results in swelling and bruising on the top and outside of the ankle, plus the usual ankle sprain symptoms.

## What's Going On in There?

Everyone twists an ankle at some point. The question is how badly it's twisted. Most common is a lateral (or inversion) sprain, where the foot rolls outward, injuring the ligaments on the outside of the ankle. The rarer medial ligament sprain is the opposite, with the foot rolling in and injuring ligaments on the inner side of the ankle.

With your basic lateral sprain, the most commonly injured ligament is the talofibular, which connects the anklebone (talus) to the smaller calf bone (fibula). More severe sprains might include the calcaneofibular ligament, which connects the fibula to the heel (calcaneus).

As with all sprains, there are three grades. Grades 1 and 2 involve varying degrees of overstretching or tearing of one or more liga-ments. A grade 3 sprain is a complete tear (rupture) of one or more ligaments.

A high-ankle sprain is different from a common ankle sprain. It usually occurs when the foot inverts (points downward) and twists, causing a stretch of the syndesmotic ligaments, which connect the tibia and fibula where your lower leg meets the top of your foot. It's called a high sprain because it happens above the ankle in the lower leg.

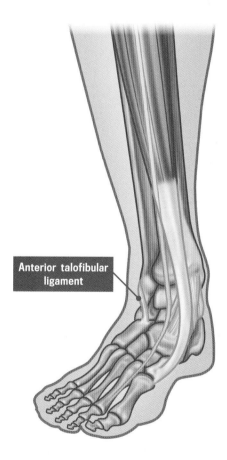

Anterior talofibular ligament

## Fix It

- **Apply first aid.** For any sprain, ice and elevation for the swelling will help (don't ice an ankle for more than 15 minutes at a time). For anything above a grade 1 sprain, crutches are a good idea. As the sprain heals, a compression bandage can help with bleeding and swelling.

- **Employ dynamic rest.** Stay fit with upper-body work. Depending on the severity of your sprain, you could try swimming or running in a pool.

- **Try an NSAID.** An anti-inflammatory like ibuprofen or naproxen can help with pain and inflammation.

- **Move it.** For simple sprains, as the pain becomes tolerable, perform basic range of motion exercises. During the first week, do only the following: Pull the foot upward, then point it away. Any side-to-side or rotating movement could aggravate the ligaments. After a week, add in rotation. With your ankle elevated, do ankle circles in either direction. Go slowly at first if the injury is still painful, but up the speed and reps as the injury heals. This will help get full range of motion back.

- **Stay flexible.** Do some simple calf stretches, as these muscles tend to tighten up to inhibit ankle movement after an injury. You don't want to strain your calf as you get back to normal activities.

## Prevent It

No one can totally prevent an ankle sprain, but you can do certain exercises to improve ankle stability, which is crucial if you've sprained your ankle once before.

- **Balance.** Simply balance on one foot. Add in complicating factors such as moving your arms, twisting your torso, and bending your knee. Also try it with your eyes closed. This is the most basic way to functionally work your ankle. (Be sure to work both sides equally to prevent imbalances.)

- **Change direction.** Run figure-8 drills, use cones for obstacle runs, or even simply draw obstacles on a driveway with chalk. The point is to challenge your lower legs and ankles in ways you don't normally to add strength and flexibility.

## When to Call a Doctor

If pain and swelling are severe, see a doctor to gauge how bad the damage is. Many things can go along with an ankle sprain—there are a lot of moving parts in the foot—including damage to the tendons, cartilage, and bones of the feet. Fractures can be common, including avulsion fractures, which occur where ligaments or tendons attach to bone.

Severe ankle injuries can include full tears (ruptures) of the talofibular and other ligaments, as well as dislocation of the ankle.

## Do You Need Surgery?

For general ankle sprains, no. But if it's a bad sprain, only a doctor can tell you. A pro needs to assess how bad your case is and what will be required to fix it (surgery, rehab, etc.).

**THE MALADY**

# Shin Splints

## The Symptoms

- **More common (roughly 90 percent of cases):** Pain in the bony part of the shin, the tibia, which hurts during and after exercise and also when you press on the area.

- **Less common (10 percent of cases):** A tightening pain in the soft, outside, muscular part of the shin. The pain is usually bad enough that running becomes impossible, and it subsides when you stop running.

## What's Going On in There?

Shin splints have derailed many an athlete's hard-won training gains. They're among the most frustrating injuries because they make the most basic act—running—impossible. But the term *shin splints* denotes more than one lower-leg ailment.

Bone-related shin pain, called medial tibial stress syndrome, can cover a broad spectrum of ailments, from a stress injury—irritation of the bone—to a stress fracture, an actual crack in the bone. It hurts during and (especially) after exercise, and the tibia hurts when touched or tapped.

Bone-related shin pain is about nine times more common than muscular shin pain; the bone actually swells and, if irritated long enough, a stress fracture can occur. It's generally the result of three variables: body mechanics, amount of activity, and bone density. Body mechanics include foot type, foot strike, and how your body is built. Activity can cause it if you up your training workload too soon. Bone

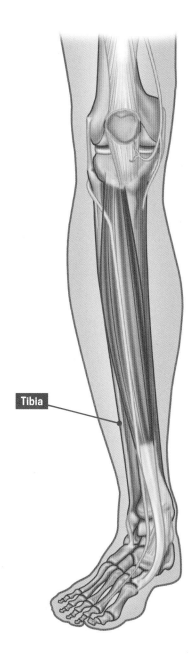

Tibia

density can be a bigger factor for women (see When to Call a Doctor). All three of these variables can be altered or adjusted to help alleviate the problem.

The less common, muscular symptoms mentioned above usually signal exertional compartment syndrome (ECS). ECS can occur in any part of the lower leg and is characterized by a tightening in the shin that worsens during exercise. Patients often report to me that their legs feel so tight they might explode. Eighty percent of ECS cases happen in the front part of the shin. The leg is pain free except during activity.

## Fix It

### BONE-RELATED:

- **See a doctor for a proper diagnosis.** Stress injuries can become stress fractures, which can sideline you for a long time.

- **Employ dynamic rest.** Find another activity that doesn't load your legs. Swimming and stationary biking are good choices.

### MUSCULAR:

- **Foam roll it.** Part of the cause of ECS is tight fascia, the tough material that wraps most of our muscles. Run your shins and calves over a foam roller for several minutes several times a day to help loosen the fascia. Manual massage can help as well.

- **Try arch supports and motion control shoes.** These can help correct biomechanical problems in the feet and take the stress off the affected muscles.

If these measures don't help, see a doctor.

## Prevent It

### BONE-RELATED:

- **Change your shoes.** Try switching to a shoe that limits pronation. Arch supports can help, as well.

- **Up your calcium and vitamin D intake.** Try 1,300 milligrams of calcium and 400 micrograms of D per day. Easy food sources are milk and yogurt.

- **Follow the 10 percent rule.** For runners, never up your weekly mileage by more than 10 percent.

- **Train your hips and core.** Strengthening these areas will make you a stronger runner, which improves foot strike and body mechanics.

- **Shorten your running stride.** Doing this while increasing your foot strike cadence may help you generate better stride mechanics because you'll be putting a lot less load on your feet, shins, knees, and on up the kinetic chain. Count your foot strikes on one side for 1 minute. A good number to shoot for is 90 strikes of one foot per minute.

### MUSCULAR:

- Foam roll and stretch (see above).

- Try arch supports and motion control shoes (see above).

## When to Call a Doctor

For bone-related pain, it's best to get a doctor's diagnosis because then you'll know the severity of the injury. You'll need an MRI to determine if a stress fracture is present, because stress fractures don't show up on an x-ray unless they're very severe or healing. Catching stress fractures early, when they're still in the stress-injury phase, is optimal. Your doctor may also do a bone density exam (using DXA, or dual-energy x-ray absorptiometry). Low bone density (osteopenia) and very low bone density (osteoporosis) have several possible causes: genetics, as these conditions tend to run in families; poor dietary calcium intake (1,300 milligrams a day is the recommended minimum); and, for women, a history of menstrual disorders, such as not getting a period for more than 6 months in a row, which can cause low levels of circulating estrogen.

## Do You Need Surgery?

Almost never. Conservative measures almost always cure bone-related shin splints. In rare cases where the bone is cracked, a rod could be installed. Also, for muscular pain, if foam rolling, massage, and footwear adjustments don't help, your doctor can test for exertional compartment syndrome by using a needle to measure the pressure inside the leg before and after exercise. When the pressure difference is high and other treatments don't work, a surgical procedure called a fasciotomy could be performed to open the fascia and give it room to expand. This procedure is rarely performed and requires 1 to 2 months of recovery.

# Runner's Knee (Patellofemoral Knee Pain)

## The Symptoms

Pain beneath the kneecap that hurts worst after you finish an activity. It's especially sore going up or down stairs, tends not to swell, and typically becomes most aggravated after about an hour of running, when your quads start to tire.

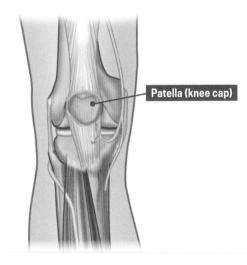

Patella (knee cap)

## What's Going On in There?

Patellofemoral knee pain—pain beneath the kneecap—is the most common type of knee pain I see in my sports medicine practice (usually about 20 cases a week). The patella (kneecap) is a sesamoid bone, which sits inside a muscle-tendon unit. In the case of the knee, the patella is located inside the patellar tendon and connects to the quadriceps muscle group, the most powerful group in the body.

The patella has to withstand tremendous amounts of force, and the direction in which the patella moves is directly related to the forces that come from the quads. For example, if an athlete has a strong lateral (or outer) quad, the patella can pull to the outer side. The back of the patella is lined with a thin layer of cartilage known as articular cartilage. This layer helps the patella track up and down along the front of the femur.

Pain can come from several causes. One is an injury to the cartilage under the patella. Poor running or biking mechanics can contribute, and that comes directly from weak or tight muscles. Poorly conditioned glutes, core

muscles, hips, and quads can lead to pelvic instability, which can affect the knees. Here's how: Ideally, your pelvis remains in a steady, level state as you run. But if your muscles are underconditioned, your pelvis will wobble as you run, the same way a car would wobble on badly aligned tires. This stresses the knees and can cause runner's knee.

I see this condition in more women than men due to what is called the Q angle, or the knock-kneed angle, which is caused by their wider hips and can result in overpronation (when the foot turns inward).

Obviously, these multiple causes of pain need to be addressed systematically to pinpoint what, exactly, the problem is. A multipronged attack as listed below can help. Once the reasons for the pain are defined, treatment is usually successful.

## Fix It

- **Employ dynamic rest.** As you work to rehab the injury, stay fit through vigorous upper-body work, plus pool running and/or biking if you can do so without knee pain.

- **Strengthen your knees, quads, and hips.** All three areas can contribute to this type of knee pain. Weak or inflexible quads are a particular problem for knee pain, but upping your strength and flexibility throughout your hips, quads, and knees will help both ease the pain and improve your form once you return to your normal training. Once you're able, plyometric lower-body exercises can help with strength and flexibility, so add multidirectional lunges, planks, skater plyos, squats, and squat jumps to your workout.

- **Work on body mechanics.** Poor running form can bring on this condition. A good way to see what your form looks like? Have a friend record you running toward a camera phone or video camera. You may see things you never realized you were doing. Do your knees fall inward? Do your feet roll inward or outward? You want your stride and foot strike to be smooth, straightforward, and neutral, which puts the least amount of stress on the knee. Increasing your strength and flexibility can help your mechanics, but you may have to concentrate on proper form or seek out a coach to help retrain you.

- **Try orthotics.** Arch supports and motion control shoes can help with overpronation (foot rolling inward).

## Prevent It

- **Rededicate yourself to strength, flexibility, and form.** All of the remedies in the Fix It section can be used as preventive measures. A good start is recording and analyzing your running form. Any improvement in your form—especially shortening your stride and raising your foot strike rate to 90 per minute—will reduce stress on crucial body parts like knees and ankles, keep your muscles from falling out of balance, and in the long run make your body less prone to breakdown.

## When to Call a Doctor

Patellofemoral knee pain is very treatable and preventable, so if pain persists after 2 months of disciplined home-based treatment or if swelling appears, you could have a different problem, and a doctor should evaluate you.

Another factor: Patients older than 50 should see a doctor for knee pain. X-rays can help diagnose patellofemoral arthritis, a wearing down of cartilage beneath the kneecap.

An MRI might be used to evaluate the cartilage in the knee joint and is often recommended if the pain hasn't subsided after 2 months of treatment or if a cartilage injury is suspected.

## Do You Need Surgery?

Almost never. The only way you run into further problems is if you don't address the pain in the first place, which could lead to cartilage and arthritis issues. But you're smart. You won't ignore your knee pain.

**THE MALADY**

# Knee Ligament Sprain

## The Symptoms

Pain at the time of the injury (usually caused by an impact) and varying pain afterward, depending on the severity of the sprain. Pain location also depends on which knee ligament is damaged. Some swelling is common, as is joint instability—feeling as if the knee might give out. Sprains are graded in severity (like strains) from grade 1 to 3.

## What's Going On in There?

There are four main ligaments in the knee that help keep the femur attached to the fibula and tibia in the lower leg. One or more of these ligaments can be sprained at the same time. However, each ligament is vulnerable to certain impacts to the knee.

- **Medial collateral ligament (MCL):** *Medial* means "inner side," so this ligament is on the inner side of the knee. This is the most commonly sprained ligament because it's vulnerable to trauma to the outside of the knee, which can easily be hit. Think of it this way: outside of knee is hit, knee bends inward, ligament on inside of knee stretches. Pain will be localized on the inside of the knee.

- **Lateral collateral ligament (LCL):** *Lateral* means "on the outer portion," so this ligament is on the outer side of the knee. This is the counterpart to the MCL. The injury process is the opposite of the MCL: inner part of knee is hit, knee bends outward,

ligament on outside of knee stretches. Pain will be localized on the outside of the knee.

- **Anterior cruciate ligament (ACL):** One of two ligaments that cross (cruciate) inside the knee joint while attaching the femur to the tibia. The anterior is the one closest to the front of the knee. It's most commonly hurt when the knee twists and the foot remains planted.

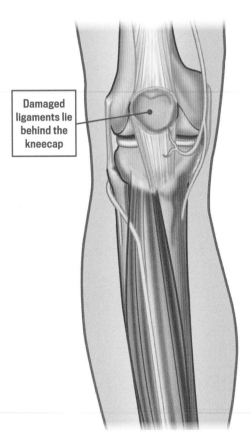

Damaged ligaments lie behind the kneecap

- **Posterior cruciate ligament (PCL):** The other crossing ligament inside the knee, it runs behind the ACL and thus is posterior. The PCL is thicker and stronger than the ACL, so it isn't injured as often. An impact on the front of the tibia while the knee is bent is the most common cause of a sprain.

### Fix It

- **See a doctor.** Don't mess around. Any knee injury needs a diagnosis. Check out When to Call a Doctor.

- **Employ dynamic rest.** Avoid loading the knee, and continue training your upper body and core.

- **Ice it.** Apply ice for 15 minutes every 4 to 6 hours during the first 2 days to alleviate swelling. Elevating the knee above your heart can also help with swelling.

- **Try NSAIDs.** Anti-inflammatories like ibuprofen and naproxen can help with pain and inflammation.

- **Rehab and strengthen.** When pain subsides and activity can resume, perform mobility and balance exercises to improve joint stability and leg strength. A good start for basic strengthening: uphill walking, cycling, or pool running. When you're pain free, build up all of your leg muscles with multidirectional lunges and squats. If you experience any pain, back off.

### Prevent It

- **Strengthen your legs.** You may never be able to prevent an impact on your knee, but the strength of your legs will help determine how badly you're hurt and how quickly you'll recover. Add a regular strength-training component to your workout regimen on top of any aerobic training that involves your legs (running, biking, etc.). Even if your knees are never injured, this training will help fend off wear and tear as you age.

### When to Call a Doctor

A mild sprain probably won't feel bad enough to drive you to a doctor—and you'll probably be okay—but any sprain symptoms should be checked out by a sports doctor. Be smart. The knee is simply too important to your future athletic performance to "suck it up" and take the pain.

Severe sprains (grade 2 or 3) won't give you a choice. You won't be able to walk, or the knee will feel like it's about to give out. Make the appointment.

The doctor will do a physical exam and any imaging (MRI etc.) that's necessary to assess total damage. The fact is, even if you suspect a sprain, you could have other damage that needs attention. These decisions and diagnoses should be made by your doctor, not you. Make the appointment.

### Do You Need Surgery?

It depends. Believe it or not, injuries to three of the four ligaments generally heal themselves. But an ACL injury needs help. Obviously this all depends on how badly you're hurt. And again, this is why it's so important to see a doctor for any knee injury.

# Torn Meniscus

### The Symptoms

Pain (especially when twisting or rotating the knee), swelling, a popping or clicking sensation, and/or stiffness in the knee. You may not be able to fully extend it. You could also have knee instability, feeling as though it will give out.

### What's Going On in There?

Each knee has a pair of menisci, C-shaped pieces of cartilage that cushion your knee between the femur and the shinbone.

Any forceful activity can lead to a torn meniscus. The most common causes: hard twisting or pivoting, sudden stops and turns, or deep squatting while lifting something heavy. Basically, any athlete is at risk of a torn meniscus, but those playing football, basketball, and tennis are especially vulnerable. Your risk increases with age, and some older adults have meniscus tears from the degeneration that occurs with age.

Oddly enough, you could have a torn meniscus and have no pain or symptoms whatsoever. Some studies peg the incidence of meniscus tear in pain-free knees between 30 and 40 percent. (Similar studies of volunteers with no back pain showed that 40 to 50 percent had herniated discs.) I have two meniscus tears myself and have no problems.

The fact is, a torn meniscus isn't necessarily a catastrophic knee injury, though it can be painful and require surgery. It's very individualized, for many instances of tears with

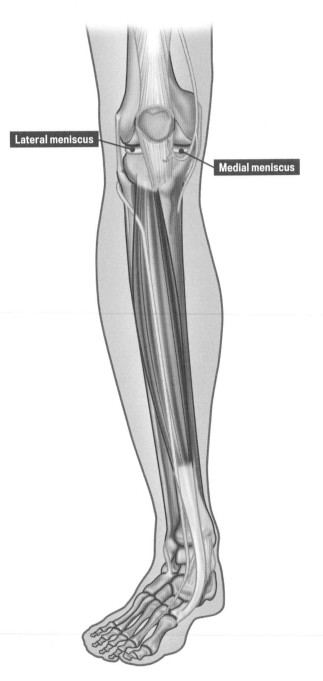

Lateral meniscus

Medial meniscus

symptoms can be treated and heal without surgery (see Fix It).

### Fix It

- **Employ dynamic rest.** Avoid loading your knee until pain and swelling subside. Concentrate on upper-body and core fitness.

- **Ice it.** Apply ice to your knee for 15 minutes every 4 to 6 hours for the first 2 days after the injury to help reduce swelling. Ice it as needed afterward.

- **Try an NSAID.** Nonsteroidal anti-inflammatories like ibuprofen and naproxen can help with pain and swelling.

- **Get back into game condition.** When you're pain free, add lower-body exercises to strengthen the leg muscles. (Squats and lunges are some of the simplest and most effective exercises.) The goal is to be stronger than you were when you originally got hurt.

### Prevent It

- **Strengthen your legs—and more.** The stronger your legs, the safer your knees. Revise your training plan to include a comprehensive lower-body and core program. Leg, knee, and hip strength are obvious goals, but a strong core will also contribute to how you move during your activity. The higher your strength and agility levels—and your core is a big part of that—the better prepared your body will be for the starts and stops that could cause a meniscus tear.

- **Wear your gear.** If your game requires knee protection, don't leave it in your gym bag.

### When to Call a Doctor

If you have symptoms, see a doctor for a proper diagnosis. Generally, a torn meniscus can be diagnosed through a physical examination of the knee. An MRI could also be used.

### Do You Need Surgery?

Here's where it can get complicated. I have had patients come in complaining of knee pain who have already had an MRI showing a meniscus tear, and they want to know if they need surgery. After examining them, I found that their knee pain was the far more common patellofemoral type (pain under the kneecap). The meniscus tear was asymptomatic.

Here's my advice: See your doctor and verify that your problems are indeed caused by a meniscus tear and not some other issue. Understand that a tear that requires surgery usually involves pain, swelling, and clicking in the knee. An MRI should be only one diagnostic tool, accompanied by a thorough physical examination. Physical therapy and home remedies can usually be options before surgery. However, if surgery is necessary, the results are generally good.

## THE MALADY

# Knee Arthritis

### The Symptoms

Pain, swelling, and stiffness in the knee and an inability to use the joint as much as one would like.

### What's Going On in There?

There are more than 100 types of arthritis, including post-infectious arthritis, which is related to infections such as Lyme disease; arthritis related to chronic disease, such as inflammatory bowel disease; and arthritis related to autoimmune disease, the most well known being rheumatoid arthritis, where the body's own immune system attacks organs and joints. Arthritis can develop in any joint, but the knees, ankles, wrists, and shoulders are common locations.

The most common form of arthritis is osteoarthritis, which affects 30 million Americans, and that number will increase in the next 20 years. It is, simply, the wearing out of a joint's lining so that bone grinds on bone. It's caused by a combination of factors, including an old injury (folks with ACL tears, for example, are 50 percent more likely to develop arthritis than folks without them), a genetic predisposition, overuse, and sometimes just bad luck.

Arthritis can get worse over time, of course. But it's also possible to continue at your current level of fitness. The strategy I recommend is to find ways to train and maintain fitness while reducing the wear and tear on your knees. Squats, climbing stairs, and

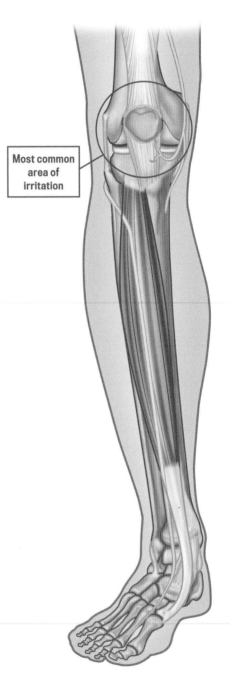

Most common area of irritation

high-mileage running are problems for folks with arthritic knees. But there are other options.

## Fix It

- **Build super legs.** Resting through arthritis, unless you're in the middle of a significant flare-up, is a bad move. More and more research shows that activity and building strength are better options. It's simple: The stronger your legs, the more you can support your knee without irritating the joint. I suggest biking and swimming to build leg strength. Quad-, hip-, and glute-strengthening exercises are also a must. Multidirectional lunges, as well as squats, squat jumps, and squat thrusts as you're able, are all good muscle builders (doing these is also a good prevention strategy).

- **Fix foot mechanics.** Pronation (foot turning inward as it strikes) puts extra pressure on the knee joint. Arch supports and motion control shoes can help relieve extra knee pounding. Also, try to shorten your stride and raise your foot strikes to 90 per minute.

- **Try supplements.** Glucosamine and chondroitin can help people with arthritis pain. You may hear mixed things about these supplements. Scientific data don't prove a definitive benefit, but many of my patients report that they have no doubt that taking them helps.

- **Try an NSAID.** Anti-inflammatories like ibuprofen and naproxen can help control pain and swelling.

- **Change the conditions.** If possible, switch to a softer running surface. Blacktop is softer than concrete, dirt and grass are softer than blacktop, and the all-weather track at your high school or local college is best of all. Your knees will thank you.

### When to Call a Doctor

If you suspect you have arthritis in your knee, it's a good idea to see a sports doctor, who can verify it easily with an x-ray. A full-on assessment of biomechanical factors such as strength, flexibility, and foot mechanics, as well as external factors such as shoe type, running surface, bike fit, and training regimen, can be a huge help.

A doctor can also administer more aggressive treatments, if warranted. For example, prescription anti-inflammatories or injectable forms of hyaluronic acid (which occurs naturally in cartilage and helps cushion joints) can help alleviate symptoms.

Last, since arthritis is degenerative, it's a good idea to establish a baseline of your condition so your doctor can continue your care and make adjustments to your activities and treatments as necessary. The goal is to stay in the game, and a sports doc can help.

### Do You Need Surgery?

Generally, no. As you get older, however, knee replacement surgery may be an option if your condition no longer responds to regular therapies.

# "Jumper's Knee" (Patellar Tendinitis)

### The Symptoms

Pain just below the kneecap and at the top of the tibia (the shinbone). The pain sharpens during leg exertion, but if the tendinitis progresses enough, any knee movement will hurt, especially going up and down stairs.

### What's Going On in There?

The patellar tendon connects your kneecap to your tibia. It's one of the main reasons you're able to extend your lower leg, whether to kick a soccer ball or jump to block a basketball.

Patellar tendinitis is a classic overuse injury. Repeated stress on the tendon causes irritation that the body can't repair fast enough, and pain results.

Anyone can get jumper's knee, but obviously it's more common in people who play jumping sports like basketball and volleyball. Also, you can irritate the patellar tendon if you increase your training load too quickly or suddenly fire up the intensity.

Ignoring the pain is a bad idea. Overusing an already overused and irritated tendon can cause tendinosis, a buildup of fluid in the tendon. Eventually, it could tear. Start treatment as soon as you feel the pain and you'll shorten both your suffering and recovery time.

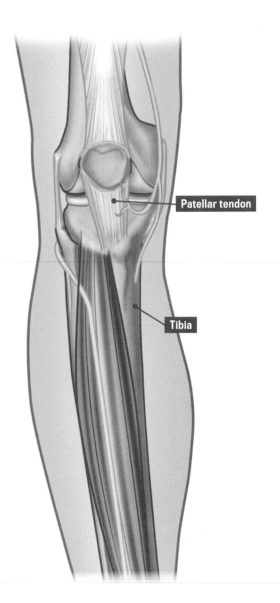

Patellar tendon

Tibia

## Fix It

- **Employ dynamic rest.** Lay off hard exertion of the knee, especially jumping. Swimming is possible if you can do it pain free. Otherwise, do intense upper-body and core workouts to maintain fitness.

- **Ice it.** Apply ice for 15 minutes several times a day to help relieve pain.

- **Try a strap.** A patellar tendon strap that goes around your leg just under the knee can offer support to the tendon and relieve pain.

- **Massage it.** Rubbing the area may help with pain and promote healing.

## Prevent It

- **Stretch your quads and hammies.** Inflexible quadriceps and hamstrings can put extra stress on the patellar tendon. Basic, disciplined stretches of both muscles can help both prevent tendinitis and heal it.

- **Try eccentric training.** Do leg extensions—however, lower the weight slowly after lifting it at normal speed. If you're rehabbing the tendon, you can first do this by having a partner apply resistance to your lower leg, then use a leg extension machine as your rehab progresses. Lowering the weight slowly challenges the tendon and the muscles around it, making it stronger. This helps prevent future cases.

**NOTE:** Normally I'm not a fan of leg extensions as a regular training exercise—they don't mimic any real-world movement and put excessive torque on the knee—but in cases of rehabbing patellar tendinitis, used as described, they can be effective.

## When to Call a Doctor

Basic conservative measures and time are usually enough to cure patellar tendinitis, depending on the severity. However, if these treatments don't help, see your doctor. He'll examine and diagnose you and, if warranted, prescribe anti-inflammatories and physical therapy.

Platelet-rich plasma (PRP) is one potential treatment. The patient's own platelets are injected into the area to speed healing. This is effective in parts of the body that have poor bloodflow and therefore heal slowly. It can be expensive and is not always covered by insurance. But for some cases, it's worth investigating.

## Do You Need Surgery?

Surgery may be an eventual option if your condition doesn't improve after 12 months. This is obviously a last resort and isn't generally needed. But if so, the surgeon can go in and repair tears in the tendon or excise damaged tissue. Recovery is 6 to 18 months, but this usually fixes the problem.

THE MALADY

# Strained/Pulled Hamstring

## The Symptoms

Tightness or pain, sometimes severe, when pressure is applied to the hamstring or when you load the muscle group.

## What's Going On in There?

The hamstring is a combination of three muscles that originate at the ischial tuberosity (the part of the pelvis you feel when you sit down) and runs along the back of the leg until it connects with bone just below the knee. Since the muscle group spans both the hip and the knee, the hamstring is subjected to two sets of forces from top to bottom—it's both a hip extensor and knee flexor.

Unfortunately, the hamstrings aren't ideally constructed for sports. The proximal hamstring (the section at the top near the hip) and the distal hamstring (the lower section near the knee) have a poor blood supply. This means slow healing rates. The middle, meaty portion of the hamstring has an excellent blood supply and heals much quicker.

When the hamstring is injured, the key is to first recognize the injury. The hamstring strain is typically the result of pushing too hard and, most importantly, not paying enough attention to pain cues.

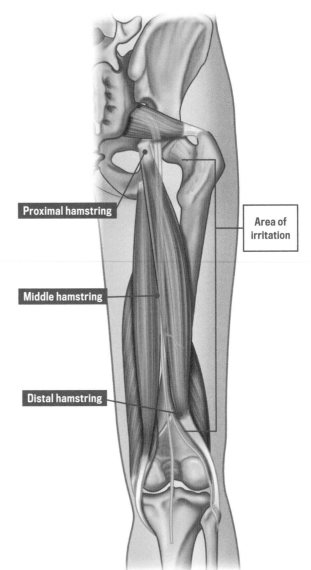

Proximal hamstring

Area of irritation

Middle hamstring

Distal hamstring

### Fix It

- **Stop.** When you feel hamstring pain, stop what you're doing. Trying to push through it will only make it worse.

- **Ice it.** Apply ice to the muscle as soon as you can after the injury, 15 minutes at a time, four to six times a day for the first 2 days.

- **Employ dynamic rest.** Avoid hamstring-loading activities, and do upper-body and core workouts to maintain fitness.

- **Stretch it—gently.** After a few days, perform gentle hamstring stretches several times a day. Depending on the severity of the strain, expect a healing time of anywhere from 2 to 8 weeks.

- **Work it—gradually.** As pain recedes, ease yourself back into activity, particularly speed and hill work. If you feel pain, don't push it. Also, use the Prevent It exercises below to rehab the muscle.

### Prevent It

- **Muscle up.** The point can't be made enough: Strong glutes, hip flexors, quads, and hamstring muscles are essential to preventing hammie pulls. Make sure squats, lunges, and planks are a regular part of your training regimen. Isolated hamstring curls can work the hamstring alone but don't help a bit with your glutes or the rest of your leg. Stick with the multimuscle exercises I mentioned for better results.

### When to Call a Doctor

Hamstring injuries generally heal after 8 weeks (for severe strains). If you still have pain after that time, see a doctor. An MRI or ultrasound can show a detailed picture of what's going on in the muscle and how much damage you have, along with any other issues you may not know about.

A sports doc can also prescribe physical therapy and other remedies. Newer treatments such as PRP (platelet-rich plasma) may offer some hope for those suffering from a lingering hamstring injury.

### Do You Need Surgery?

Hamstring surgery is rare but not unheard of, and it is only used to repair significant tears or ruptures. If that's your problem, trust me, you'll know it.

**THE MALADY**

# Proximal Hamstring Strain (aka "Pain in the Butt")

### The Symptoms

Discomfort in the gluteus muscle, especially during the push-off phase of running and other sports. The harder you push, the harder it grabs.

### What's Going On in There?

Gluteal pain can signal several injuries—a strained glute or piriformis muscle, or inflammation of the sciatic nerve—but this pain, especially when associated with the push-off phase of running, is a hamstring strain.

The hamstring, a set of three muscles running from your ischial tuberosity (the pelvis bones you feel when you sit down) down the back of your leg to just below the knee, is divided into three sections. The distal hamstring is the lower section near the knee; the middle hamstring is the meaty part in the middle; and the proximal hamstring, the upper section near the hip. The "pain in the butt" hamstring strain is a proximal hamstring strain and presents its own difficulties, different than those posed by the lower hamstring strains.

Strains come from overuse, pushing the muscle too hard, or weakness in the surrounding muscles. A mild strain begins as a dull ache in the buttock and, if not treated, progresses to a sharp pain that prohibits using your leg with any power.

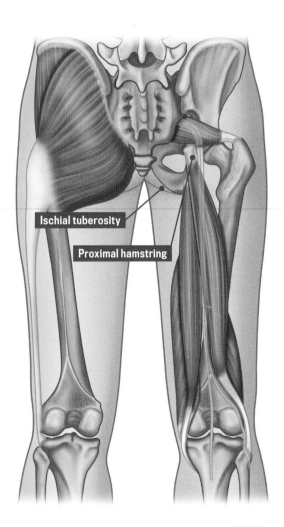

Ischial tuberosity

Proximal hamstring

What's worse, the proximal hamstring has a lousy blood supply, which means it generally takes longer to heal than other hamstring strains might.

## Fix It

- **Stop.** As soon as you feel gluteal pain, stop your athletic activity immediately. If you try to push through the pain, you'll make the injury worse.

- **Employ dynamic rest.** Avoid hamstring-loading activities, and do upper-body and core workouts to maintain fitness.

- **Ice it.** Apply ice to the muscle as soon as you can after the injury, 15 minutes at a time, four to six times a day for the first 2 days.

- **Stretch it—gently.** After a few days, perform gentle hamstring stretches several times a day. Depending on the severity of the strain, expect a healing time of anywhere from 2 to 8 weeks. More severe strains could take longer.

- **Work it—gradually.** As pain recedes, ease yourself back into activity, particularly speed and hill work. If you feel pain, don't push it.

## Prevent It

- **Strengthen your glutes and core.** A weak butt creates muscle activation problems for the muscles that come off the pelvis. For the glutes, it's squats, squats, and more squats: single-leg squats, jumping plyometric squats, squat thrusts, or similar exercises. Do these at least three times a week.

For the core, which helps pelvic stability, do 5 to 6 minutes of planks per day. It's simple, but it makes an incredible difference in injury prevention.

- **Shorten your stride.** For distance runners, shortening your stride can reduce stress on the hamstring.

- **Check the fit of your bike.** For cyclists, checking the fit of your bike—specifically, the height of your seat—can help. A high seat puts more stress on the hamstring.

## When to Call a Doctor

If a tincture of time and gradual stretching and activity don't fix the problem after 8 weeks, see a doctor. An ultrasound or MRI can identify a severe injury or tear. A sports doc can give a more targeted prescription based on your individual case, including a physical therapy plan that can deliver rehab, as well as a progressive program of stretching and strengthening to get you back to normal activity.

The key to any hamstring treatment, whether home based or guided by a physician, is making sure you don't try to do too much too soon. Conservative is always the way to go, and in the meantime, work other areas of your body to stay fit.

## Do You Need Surgery?

Hamstring surgery is rare but not unheard of, and it is only used to repair significant tears or ruptures. If that's your problem, trust me, you'll know it.

# Post-Workout Quad and/or Glute Soreness

## The Symptoms

General muscle soreness, especially the day after an intense workout or starting a new activity. However, delayed-onset muscular soreness, a specific and serious condition, can be incredibly painful.

## What's Going On in There?

When muscle tissue is injured from exercise, the fibers tear. Ideally, in a day or two, the fibers repair themselves and are stronger than before. This is the basis of building muscle, and normal muscle soreness after a workout—especially in the first few weeks of intensified activity—is to be expected.

If your muscle soreness is intense and doesn't present itself until 24 to 48 hours after the muscle injury, however, you may have a serious condition called delayed-onset muscle soreness (DOMS). It can happen from excessive loading force on muscle cells. It's important to distinguish the symptoms of DOMS from the everyday aches and pains that come after hard exercise. This pain can be severe.

Why is DOMS serious? When muscle tissue is injured, a process called *rhabdomyolysis* causes it to release a protein called *myoglobin*. We all have a bit of myoglobin release after hard athletic events. Several studies have looked at healthy athletes after marathons and found mild to moderate

amounts of myoglobin in the urine, a condition called *myoglobinuria*. When the muscle injury is more serious, however, the amounts of myoglobin can be quite high. The urine can be dark colored—which is a big red flag—and in some cases kidney damage and even kidney failure can result.

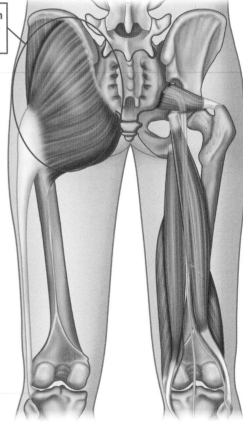

Most common area of glute soreness

## Fix It

**NORMAL POST-WORKOUT SORENESS:**

- **Hydrate, fuel up, sleep well.** Give your body the best opportunity to repair muscle damage and come back strong. Drink fluids until your urine is clear, eat smart, and get a great night's sleep. The best restoration and recovery happen while you sleep.

- **Try an NSAID.** Anti-inflammatories like ibuprofen or naproxen can help alleviate soreness.

**DELAYED-ONSET MUSCLE SORENESS:**

- **Hydrate and see your doctor.** If you suspect you have DOMS, start drinking lots of fluids and call your doctor. A sports doctor is a better bet and will have more experience identifying DOMS.

## Prevent It

- **Hydrate.** Proper hydration before any exercise or athletic event can help ease common post-exercise muscle soreness and, more importantly, prevent DOMS. Factors to consider: temperature and humidity (Vegas versus Seattle); your planned intensity (race pace versus easy run); overall health the previous week (even a mild stomach bug or

diarrhea can dehydrate you). Drink enough fluids to keep your urine running clear.

## When to Call a Doctor

If your muscle pain and soreness are severe, seemed to come on 24 to 48 hours after hard activity, and your urine is dark, see your doctor immediately.

Your doctor will do a urinalysis to check myoglobin levels and, if necessary, perform blood tests to determine if there's been any kidney damage.

DOMS is much more common than most athletes realize. Why some athletes experience DOMS and others don't is not yet understood, but one of the most important factors is dehydration before, during, and after an intense activity. Some athletes just seem prone to developing DOMS and get it often, probably because of biological and genetic factors affecting their muscle tissue.

The good news: DOMS is usually preventable with smart pre-exercise behavior and athlete education.

## Do You Need Surgery?

No.

# Strained Quad

### The Symptoms

Anything from a twinge to a sharp pain in the thigh, depending on the severity of the strain. Trying to straighten the leg against resistance causes pain. Swelling and bruising are possible. For a grade 2 or 3 strain, the pain affects walking.

### What's Going On in There?

The quadriceps group, at the front, upper part of the leg, includes a set of four muscles (thus, "quads"): vastus lateralis, vastus medialis, vastus intermedius, and rectus femoris. The latter is the most commonly strained quad muscle because it runs from the hip to the knee and crosses both joints and, thus, faces double jeopardy (hip and knee stress). However, the most common site of a strain is the point where muscle turns to tendon just above the knee.

Sprinting, jumping, or kicking are usually the causes, though any movement can cause a strain.

### Fix It

- **Employ dynamic rest.** Avoid loading the leg, especially in the acute stage (first 48 to 72 hours, depending on the severity). Concentrate on upper-body and core work to maintain fitness.

- **Ice it.** Apply ice for 15 minutes four to six times a day for the first 2 days.

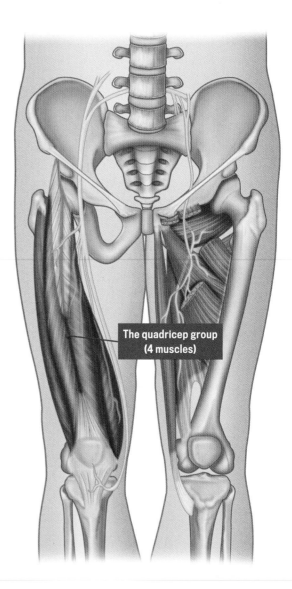

The quadricep group (4 muscles)

- **Compress and elevate.** A compression bandage and elevating the leg can help with swelling and inflammation.

- **Stretch it—gently.** After several days, if it's comfortable, perform gentle quad stretches (for 20 to 30 seconds) several times a day. Also do hip flexor stretches: Kneel with the knee on the strained side on the floor and the other leg out front with knee bent (sort of like a lunge, but with the back knee on the ground). With your back straight, push your hips forward until you feel the stretch in the hip and thigh. Hold for 20 to 30 seconds for 3 reps several times a day.

- **Strengthen it—gradually.** Three quad exercises work well for rebuilding the injured muscle. Ease into them slowly and do only as many reps as comfort allows. As time goes on, you should be able to do them more easily and with more intensity. For the straight-leg raise, sit on the floor with your back straight and your legs straight out in front of you. Slowly raise one leg, keeping it straight, hold for a second, and then lower it. The other two exercises are more common: lunges and squats. For single-leg exercises, be sure to do equal reps with both legs to avoid a muscle imbalance.

### Prevent It

- See the stretching and strengthening exercises under Fix It to reinforce your quads against injury.

### When to Call a Doctor

For a severe strain (if walking is difficult) or if you don't get relief from pain through home-based treatment for milder strains, see a doctor.

A sports doc can use MRIs and x-rays to determine the extent and specifics of your injury. A doctor or physical therapist can prescribe ultrasound or electrostimulation, plus sports massage techniques, along with stretching and strengthening exercises.

### Do You Need Surgery?

Generally, no.

# Strained Glute

## The Symptoms

A sharp pain or pulling in the glutes, the intensity depending on the grade of the strain. In mild cases, the pain can increase after the activity but doesn't make you stop doing it. More severe strains could have you limping off the field immediately. Running, jumping, and lunging cause pain, but you'll also feel pain walking up or down stairs, walking uphill, and possibly even sitting.

## What's Going On in There?

Three muscles make up the gluteal group: the gluteus maximus, gluteus medius, and gluteus minimus. They connect on the pelvis and the femur. They help stabilize the pelvis and are integral in running, jumping, squatting, and lunging.

Strains most commonly occur when the muscles contract while in the middle of a stretch. Examples: sudden acceleration while running, doing weighted squats in a gym, or jumping. Naturally, athletes in football, basketball, track and field, and soccer are prime candidates for glute strains. They also can occur during weight training. The older you are and the less you warm up before an activity, the greater your strain risk.

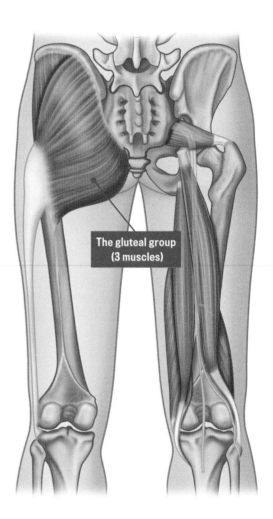

The gluteal group
(3 muscles)

## Fix It

- **Employ dynamic rest.** Avoid running, jumping, lunging, and stairs. Upper-body work and swimming are good if you can do them pain free.

- **Ice it.** Apply ice for 15 minutes every 4 to 6 hours for the first 2 days.

- **Try an NSAID.** Anti-inflammatories like ibuprofen and naproxen can help with swelling and inflammation.

- **Stretch and strengthen your glutes.** When you can perform these simple exercises without too much discomfort, start slow and gradually increase until you can do a set of 10 to 20 reps three times a day.

  - *Gluteal stretch:* Lie on your back. Bring one knee to your chest and use your hands to pull the knee toward your opposite shoulder. Hold for several seconds and repeat. Do both sides even if only one side is injured.

  - *Gluteal bridge:* Lie on your back with your knees raised and feet flat on the floor. With your hands and arms braced flat on the floor, raise your hips until your knees, hips, and shoulders are in a straight line. You should feel your glutes flex. Hold for several seconds, lower, and repeat.

  - *Chair squat:* Stand in front of a chair and do a squat while holding on to the chair, then stand. Work your way up to 6 sets of 15 reps. Then do one-legged chair squats, up to several sets of 15 reps on each leg. All of this will get you strong enough to do squats without the chair.

## Prevent It

- **Work your core, hips, and hamstrings.** Your glutes work very closely with that entire system of muscles—as they form a big part of the kinetic chain—and weakness or instability in one or more of those areas can affect how your glutes perform. Squats, lunges, and planks are all must-do exercises to help the biggest muscles in your body play nice with all their friends around them.

## When to Call a Doctor

In the case of a grade 3 strain (rupture), you'll have no choice. But for less severe cases, 2 to 6 weeks is the general time frame for healing. If pain persists, see a sports doctor.

Physical therapy including ultrasound and electrostimulation can help heal the muscle. In the case of a rupture, surgery may be required. In that case, you generally will be out of action for 6 months or more.

## Do You Need Surgery?

Generally, no. Surgery is rare.

## THE MALADY

# Strained Adductor (Groin Strain)

### The Symptoms

Pain in the inner thigh close to the groin. Pain can be sharp and severe for sudden injuries, or a dull ache getting worse over time for minor strains that become chronic because you "play through the pain." The level of pain depends on the grade of the strain.

### What's Going On in There?

The adductor is a collection of muscles running from the groin down along the inside of the femur. They help you move side to side, as well as bring your knees together.

Injuries most often occur during an explosive change of direction or side-to-side movement, as well as during sudden acceleration in a sprint. Kicking and twisting of the leg can also be a factor, which means that virtually all athletes are at risk.

Even worse risk factors: weakness and lack of flexibility in the adductor group. As with any muscle group, if it isn't trained for the job requirement, it will fail when put to the test (see Prevent It for strengthening strategies).

A good way to determine if your injury is an adductor strain and not some other hip injury (strained hip flexor, for example) is to try moving your knee inward toward the other knee against resistance. Pain in the inner thigh is your main clue. Depending on the grade of the strain, expect healing time to range from a few days to more than a month, though grade 3 strains will require more time and a doctor's care (see When to Call a Doctor).

### Fix It

■ **Employ dynamic rest.** Avoid lower-body movement that will aggravate the adductor. Use upper-body workouts to maintain fitness. You can also work your core, but be careful to avoid any movements that cause pain in the injured area—the hips and core work together in many movements.

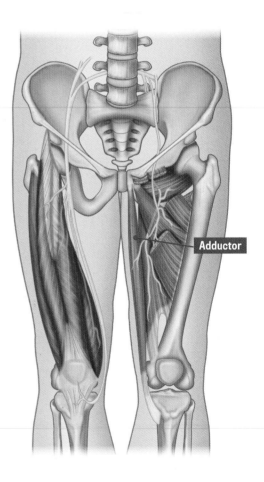

Adductor

- **Ice it.** Apply ice for 15 minutes every 4 to 6 hours for the first 2 days.

- **Try an NSAID.** Anti-inflammatories like ibuprofen and naproxen can help with swelling and inflammation.

- **Stretch it.** When you can do so with little or no pain, begin basic stretching and strengthening exercises. Try these.
  - *Sitting groin stretch:* Sit on the floor with your knees bent and the bottoms of your feet pressed together. Press the tops of your knees down toward the floor with your elbows. Hold for 10 to 15 seconds, then release. Repeat 3 to 5 times.
  - *Standing groin stretch:* Stand with your legs shoulder-width apart. Shift your weight to one side, bending your knee slightly. Stop when you feel a stretch in your adductor, then hold for 10 to 15 seconds. Return to the starting position and repeat 3 to 5 times.

- **Strengthen it.** When you can do so with little or no pain, do side and diagonal lunges, which are standard lunges except that you do them to each side, as well as diagonally to each side and behind. Do a set of 5 in each direction, upping your reps and sets as you get stronger and become completely pain free.

## Prevent It

- **Train your groin.** The best prevention is a strong and supple set of adductors. Core work, multidirectional lunges, squats, and squat jumps should be staples of your lower-body work (yes, your core works with your adductors). Add in skater plyos, which are explosive side lunges that mimic the motion of a speed skater. Also useful: If you have access to one, a lateral slide board (where you wear special sliding socks over your sneakers) gives your adductors a terrific workout.

## When to Call a Doctor

Understand that the adductor muscles have a lousy blood supply and an abundant nerve supply, which means an injury will be painful and take longer to heal than other muscle strains. Home-based self-care as described here is usually effective, though expect complete healing in weeks rather than days. Platelet-rich plasma (PRP) injections have been used successfully and could be an option in cases that don't respond to conservative measures.

Severe strains, however, need medical attention. Any loss of function, as when you have difficulty bringing one knee closer to the other, signals a severe tear or rupture. You'll need imaging (MRI and/or ultrasound) and a diagnosis to determine just how much damage there is and if it involves muscles, tendons, or both, as well as whether there is any nerve involvement.

## Do You Need Surgery?

Surgery is a real possibility in the worst cases (though it's not guaranteed) and, if needed, will probably keep you out of action for 3 to 6 months. However, with proper rehab and strengthening, patients usually have a full recovery.

## THE MALADY

# Piriformis Syndrome

### The Symptoms

Pain in the lower back and/or buttocks, sometimes feeling as if it's deep inside the buttock muscles. Sometimes it can be too painful to sit on the affected buttock. The pain and/or tingling can radiate down the backs of the legs as well.

### What's Going On in There?

The piriformis muscle runs behind the hip joint and aids in external hip rotation, or turning your leg outward. The catch here is that the piriformis crosses over the sciatic nerve. The piriformis muscle can become tight from, for example, too much sitting (a problem many working people can relate to). The muscle can also be strained or spasm from overuse. In piriformis syndrome, this tightness or spasm causes the muscle to compress and irritates the sciatic nerve. This brings on lower-back and buttock pain, sometimes severe. The diagnosis is tricky because piriformis syndrome can very easily be confused with sciatica.

The difference in diagnosis is that traditional sciatica is generally caused by some spinal issue, like a compressed lumbar disc. Piriformis syndrome becomes the go-to diagnosis when sciatica is present with no discernible spinal cause.

Runners, cyclists, and rowers are the most at-risk athletes for piriformis syndrome. They engage in pure forward movement, which can weaken hip adductors and abductors, the

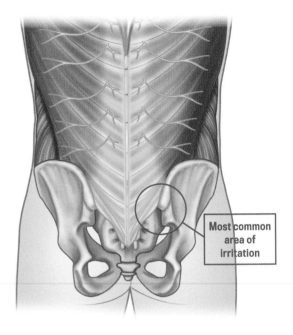

Most common area of irritation

muscles that allow us to open and close our legs. Throw in some weak glutes, and all those poorly conditioned muscles put extra strain on the piriformis. And you've got a painful problem.

Another risk for runners: Overpronating (foot turning inward) can cause the knee to rotate on impact. The piriformis fires to help prevent the knee from rotating too much, which can lead to overuse and tightening of the muscle.

### Fix It

■ **Employ dynamic rest.** Stop the offending activity (if your pain is moderate to severe, you'll want to anyway). Use upper-body workouts to maintain fitness. Core work will probably be a problem, as your lower back and glutes will hurt. Let the pain be your guide, and back off immediately if anything hurts.

- **Try an NSAID.** Anti-inflammatories like ibuprofen and naproxen can help with swelling and inflammation.

- **Stretch your hip rotators.** As pain allows, try to gradually open up your hips by stretching your hip flexors and rotators. These two stretches can help.

  - *Seated piriformis stretch:* While sitting in a chair with your back straight, rest your right ankle on your left knee. Then gently press down on your right knee until you feel a stretch in your hips. Hold for 10 to 15 seconds. Repeat several times and for the opposite hip.

  - *Lying piriformis stretch:* Lie on your back with your knees raised and feet flat on the floor. Put your right ankle on your left knee. Raise your left foot while pressing down on your right knee until you feel the stretch in your hip and buttock. Hold for 10 to 15 seconds. Repeat several times and for the opposite hip.

## Prevent It

- **Stretch and strengthen.** As with many of the interconnected muscles in this region of the body, each supports the other, and weakness in one area can mess up the works. In short, if you want a healthy piriformis, you need a strong core, glutes,

hips, and legs. That means lots of core work, multidirectional lunges, squats, squat jumps, and skater plyos. Also add some hip-specific exercises at least once a week. Try the dirty dog. While on all fours, lift your right leg outward (like a dog would do by a fire hydrant), hold for a second, and lower. Do a couple sets of 10 reps per leg. You can also add in a hip rotation to this move when you lift your leg.

- **Try orthotics.** Motion control shoes and over-the-counter arch supports can help overpronation and reduce the chain reaction between the knee and piriformis.

## When to Call a Doctor

If home-based care doesn't improve your symptoms in a week (or sooner if the pain is severe), see a doctor. A sports doctor may continue with conservative treatments like those mentioned here, but you'll also have a thorough examination to confirm the diagnosis, which, as I mentioned, can be tricky, given the similarity to sciatica. Also, a doctor may prescribe muscle relaxers that could be more effective than over-the-counter NSAIDs.

If conservative treatments fail, your doctor could opt for injections. A local anesthetic (lidocaine), corticosteroids, or even Botox— or a combination of them—can be used. The injection is tricky because of how deep the piriformis is in the hip, but the results are generally good.

## Do You Need Surgery?

Surgery is very rare.

# Abdominal Strain

### The Symptoms

A sharp pain in your torso at the injury site. You'll really feel it during any muscle flexion, including breathing deeply, coughing, sneezing, or laughing.

### What's Going On in There?

Your abdominal muscles (which are much more than simply "abs") run in layers across and around your trunk. There are four main components.

- **Transverse abdominis.** These are the deepest layer of abdominals; they keep everything that's inside from finding its way outside. These muscle fibers run horizontally across your front, protect your vital organs, and help you laugh, cough, and sneeze.

- **Internal and external obliques.** These muscles run diagonally along your sides and help with trunk rotation. For more on them, see Oblique Strain on page 106.

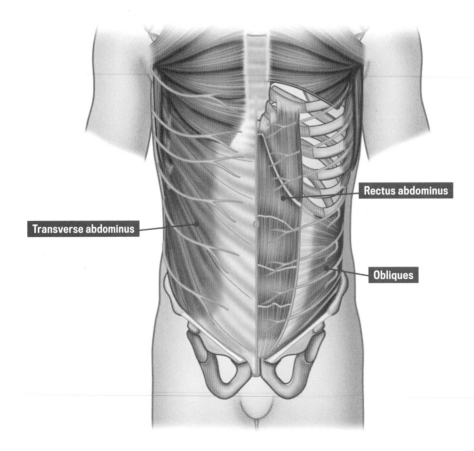

Transverse abdominus

Rectus abdominus

Obliques

- **Rectus abdominis.** These run vertically, closest to the skin. Yes, these form your legendary six-pack. They also aid in trunk flexion.

Like any strain, an abdominal strain comes in three grades, 1 to 3, with 3 being a complete rupture. Grade 1 is pretty straightforward: The area hurts, especially when the muscle is engaged, but you can function. Once you get into grade 2 territory, you could have swelling and bruising, and you'll find most movements excruciating. Grade 3? You'll be incapacitated and need emergency care.

Any activity requiring explosive trunk rotation or flexion puts you at risk.

### Fix It

- **Employ dynamic rest.** An abdominal strain is a very frustrating injury because our core is so integral to so many movements. Avoid any activity that activates your core. To stay fit, try lower-body workouts that keep muscle flexion below the waist. As long as you can do it pain free, jogging and stationary cycling, as well as multidirectional lunges, can work.

- **Ice it.** Apply ice for 15 minutes every 4 to 6 hours for the first 2 days.

- **Try an NSAID.** Anti-inflammatories like ibuprofen and naproxen can help with swelling and inflammation.

- **Rehab it.** Once you're pain free, return low-intensity ab work to your workout.

Bridges and planks are great for this, but be careful not to overdo it early on. When you're able to return to full activity, be sure to intensify your core work so you're stronger than when you were injured (see Prevent It).

### Prevent It

- **Build a powerful core.** The bottom line: Strains happen because the muscle can't handle what you ask of it. Make the muscle stronger and more flexible. Core-specific training must be a serious part of your workout regimen. Incorporate trunk rotation, use resistance, and stretch. I also recommend regular Pilates classes.

### When to Call a Doctor

If the pain doesn't improve in 2 weeks, make an appointment. Depending on the severity, ab strains generally heal within 2 to 8 weeks, but you should see some improvement after 2; if not, a doctor can evaluate the severity of your injury and any other underlying factors.

More aggressive treatments could include ultrasound therapy, corticosteroid injections, or physical therapy.

### Do You Need Surgery?

Almost never. The most severe ruptures could require surgery—and you'll know it. If you have a full-blown rupture, trust me, you'll want to go to the ER immediately.

# Oblique Strain

### The Symptoms

A sharp pain in the side between the lower ribs and the hips. Pain can be severe and increases when the muscle is stretched or contracted by leaning to the left or right (depending on which side is hurt).

### What's Going On in There?

The obliques are part of your core and run down the side of your body from your lower ribs to your hips. The internal obliques are deeper than your external obliques and work with your rectus abdominis muscles to help you twist and bend. Whereas the rectus abdominis fibers run vertically and transverse abdominis ones run horizontally, the oblique fibers run diagonally (though in opposite directions). The internal and external obliques also complement each other on opposite sides. Example: If you twist your torso to the left, your left internal oblique and right external oblique work together to

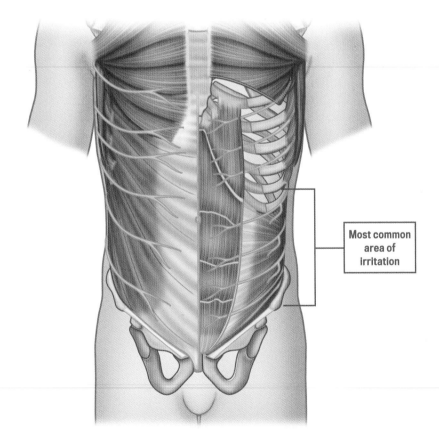

Most common
area of
irritation

make it happen, and vice versa if you twist to the right.

Any forceful twisting or overuse can injure your obliques, so baseball and softball players, golfers, tennis players, and any other swing-centric athletes are at risk. Oblique injuries can be easily aggravated, so they can nag if not properly treated.

As with all strains, oblique strains range from grade 1 to 3, with 3 being a complete tear or rupture.

### Fix It

- **Employ dynamic rest.** An oblique strain is a touchy injury because our core is so integral to so many movements and it's very easy to aggravate it. Avoid any activity that activates your core, especially any twisting movements. To stay fit, try lower-body workouts that keep muscle flexion below the waist. As long as you can do it pain free, jogging and stationary cycling, as well as multidirectional lunges, can work.

- **Ice it.** Apply ice for 15 minutes every 4 to 6 hours for the first 2 days.

- **Try an NSAID.** Anti-inflammatories like ibuprofen and naproxen can help with swelling and inflammation.

- **Rehab it.** Once you're pain free, return low-intensity ab work to your workout. Bridges and planks are great for this, and you can also add in rotational ab exercises

and side planks, but be careful not to overdo it early on. When you're able to return to full activity, be sure to intensify your rotational core work so you're stronger than when you were injured (see Prevent It).

### Prevent It

- **Build a twisting, turning core.** The bottom line: Strains happen because the muscle can't handle what you ask of it. Make your obliques stronger and more flexible. Core-specific training must be a serious part of your workout regimen. Incorporate trunk rotation, use resistance, and stretch. I also recommend regular Pilates classes.

### When to Call a Doctor

If the pain doesn't improve in 2 weeks, make an appointment. Depending on the severity, oblique strains generally heal within 2 to 8 weeks, but you should see some improvement after 2; if not, a doctor can evaluate the severity of your injury and any other underlying factors.

More aggressive treatments could include ultrasound therapy, corticosteroid injections, or physical therapy.

### Do You Need Surgery?

Almost never. The most severe ruptures could require surgery—and you'll know it. If you have a full-blown rupture, trust me, you'll want to go to the ER immediately.

# Side Stitch

### The Symptoms

A sharp pain in the side while running, sometimes severe enough to force you to stop.

### What's Going On in There?

The dreaded side stitch can be caused by several things. The most common cause is a diaphragm spasm—especially for runners just starting out or pushing a run beyond their current capability. The diaphragm is the muscle that separates the lungs and chest cavity from the abdominal cavity, and it expands and contracts with every breath. When it works too hard, it can spasm, causing a pain that feels like a knife in your side.

Another common scenario: The diaphragm is working fine, but the breathing effort is excessive due to panting and puffing, and the accessory muscles of breathing, the obliques, spasm.

Other causes that are less common include

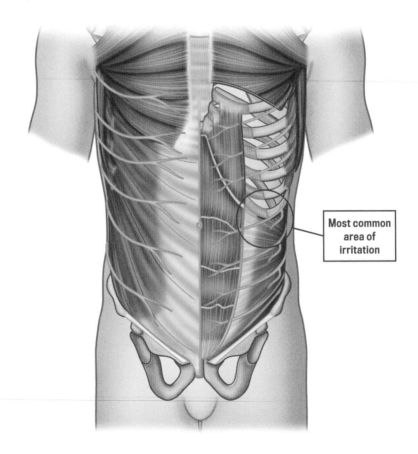

Most common
area of
irritation

exercise-induced bronchospasm (EIB) and an anatomical problem with the lungs.

Triathletes face a cause specific to their sport—the stress of transitioning from cycling to running. If the core muscles aren't stretched after a long cycling leg, they may spasm.

### Fix It

■ **Stretch it.** First, try to relieve the side stitch without stopping your run. Raise your arm on the side that hurts and place your hand on the back of your head. Continue running. The idea is to allow those side muscles to stretch, hopefully relieving the spasm and, of course, the pain. Try this for 30 seconds to a minute. Repeat if the side stitch returns or doesn't abate.

If this is ineffective, take a break and stretch those side muscles as you rest. This is a two-pronged attack. One, you stretch the spasming muscles. And two, you rest your diaphragm and obliques, which should solve the problem.

### Prevent It

■ **Strengthen your core.** Since the most common causes of side stitches are muscle related, increasing core strength through exercises like planks and crunches, especially with rotation, often fixes the problem.

### When to Call a Doctor

If you get chronic side stitches and none of these basic measures works, see a sports doctor. Your side stitches could be lung related, caused by exercise-induced bronchospasm (EIB) or an anatomical problem with the lungs. If that's your diagnosis, your doctor will most likely prescribe an inhaler, which is usually effective in these cases. (However, your author/doctor says with a smile, it's still a good idea to keep your core strong. Planks and core rotation, kids!)

### Do You Need Surgery?

No.

**THE MALADY**

# Lower-Back Spasms (Muscular Back Pain)

### The Symptoms

Muscular back pain usually comes on instantly. Pain radiates out from both sides of the spine, and the muscles feel like they're locked up. It can be severe and debilitating.

### What's Going On in There?

Muscular back pain is the most common type of back pain. It involves the paraspinal muscles, also known as the erector spinae muscle group, strong muscles on either side of the spine that are responsible for moving, twisting, and bending the spine. These muscles run from the back of the hip along the spine and all the way up to the bottom of the skull. They're among the strongest muscles in the body.

So what brings on the pain? In general, the paraspinal muscles are either too tight or too weak—or both. A sudden twisting or wrenching can set it off, as can bending forward or even a direct impact on the muscle. Acute muscular back pain can be excruciating.

Other muscle groups can also contribute to back pain. If you have weak or tight hamstrings, core muscles, glutes, or hip flexors, it could affect body alignment, mechanics, or other factors that could force your back muscles to compensate and overextend themselves.

### Fix It

- **Employ dynamic rest.** Bad back spasms will make you want to lie down for, oh,

several years or so. Don't. Don't even lie down for an afternoon. Stay mobile, even if it means taking little shuffle steps around the house. Bed rest during spells of back pain only deconditions your muscles, which is the opposite of what you want to happen. During the acute stage, avoid straining your back, but do simple stretches to loosen your hamstrings, hip flexors, and glutes. All of these can help alleviate the spasm.

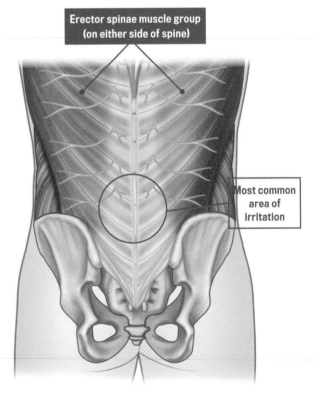

Erector spinae muscle group (on either side of spine)

Most common area of irritation

- **Ice it, then heat it.** Apply ice for 15 minutes every 4 to 6 hours for the first 2 days. After 48 hours, a heating pad at the same time intervals can help relieve the spasms.

- **Try an NSAID.** Anti-inflammatories like ibuprofen and naproxen can help with pain and inflammation.

- **Vary your therapies.** Back pain therapies are very individualized. For example, some of my patients respond well to massage therapy. Others swear by acupuncture. Chiropractic can help as well, though your treatment should be for only a designated time frame and include a fitness and flexibility component. My point: Try different therapies until you get results. Everyone responds differently to different things.

- **Stretch and strengthen your kinetic chain.** As the pain subsides, start the reconditioning process with basic core-strengthening and stretching exercises. Go slow. Stretch your hamstrings, hip flexors, glutes, and core. Do glute bridges and planks, adding reps and intensity as you improve. Once you're pain free, up your kinetic chain conditioning (see Prevent It).

## Prevent It

- **Commit to your kinetic chain.** Back pain prevention isn't just about strengthening your back muscles. Your back is working in combination with your entire core, glutes, hips, hamstrings, and quads for optimal performance. Your fitness program must include dynamic, compound exercises that target as many of these areas as possible. Workout staples should include multidirec-

tional lunges, core exercises with trunk rotation, squats, squat jumps, burpees, planks, mountain climbers, and more. Plyometric total-body boot-camp-style workouts are terrific. I also recommend regular Pilates classes. All of these things focus on strength and flexibility throughout your kinetic chain, especially your core. Again, back pain prevention isn't just about your back muscles.

## When to Call a Doctor

In general, muscular back pain doesn't require a doctor's visit, but depending on how bad your pain is, it could be a good idea. Doctors see a lot of these cases, so you'll get a thorough going-over to ensure there are no underlying issues beyond muscle spasms (osteoarthritis and spinal stenosis, to name two).

X-rays can rule out bone issues, and an MRI can illuminate disc issues, though that may not be helpful. Herniated lumbar discs can show up yet have nothing to do with your back pain (studies have shown that 30 to 40 percent of folks with no back pain whatsoever have herniated discs).

A doctor can also prescribe muscle relaxers, which can help alleviate the spasm and allow you to begin rehabbing.

## Do You Need Surgery?

No. Muscular back pain almost always improves with these conservative home-based measures. One helpful hint: Never forget how painful back spasms can be; it's a great motivator to keep your core in top condition to prevent another flare-up.

# Muscular Neck Pain

### The Symptoms

Pain, sometimes severe, in the muscles of your neck that can cause a spasm or "locking up" sensation.

### What's Going On in There?

The human body has a set of muscles that run on both sides of your spine all the way up from your tailbone to the back of your head. That's a lot of muscle. And that's why muscular pain is the most common type of neck pain.

Localized pain is the main giveaway that your problem is muscular—a much simpler issue to treat—and not something related to your cervical spine (your upper spine, including the neck). When you get muscle spasms on the sides of your neck, the pain tends not to radiate down into your fingers like it would with a cervical disc or nerve problem—see Nerve-Based Neck Pain (Cervical Radiculopathy) on page 114. The pain is in the muscles on one or both sides of your spine and that's it.

The causes are usually classic: asking too much of an unprepared or fatigued muscle, overuse, or even sleeping in the wrong position.

### Fix It

- **Employ dynamic rest.** Avoid any activities that engage the neck and shoulders. Use lower-body workouts to maintain fitness.

- **Ice it.** Apply ice to the neck for 15 minutes four to six times a day for the first 48 hours.

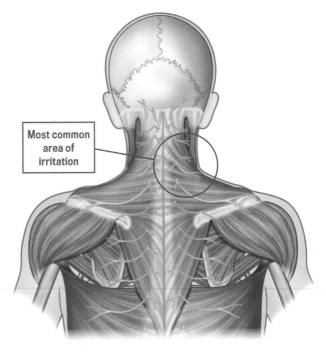

Most common area of irritation

- **Try an NSAID.** Anti-inflammatories like ibuprofen and naproxen can help with swelling and inflammation.

- **Go for a massage.** Massaging and basic stretching of the neck muscles can help a lot. A professional massage therapist will be trained in addressing this type of pain.

- **Reestablish range of motion.** As pain improves, try these exercises to help recondition your neck and shoulders. Once you're pain free, move on to more aggressive neck and shoulder conditioning to help prevent the problem from recurring.

- *Neck stretches:* Stand with your hands behind your neck. Bend your neck back and look at the ceiling. Squeeze your shoulder blades together. Hold for a second and return to the starting position. Work up to 10 reps. Also try basic head rotation, to the left and right, as well as tilting your head to the side, left and right, for up to 10 reps each.

- *Basic resistance:* Do the same movements in the above stretches, but change them to resistance exercises by using your hands to prevent your head from moving; i.e., put your hand on the right side of your head and try to tilt your head to the right while your hand prevents it. Hold for 5 seconds. Do this for left and right tilt, left and right head turn, and forward and backward movements.

- *Shoulder rehab:* Shoulder shrugs, holding at the top for 5 seconds, are effective. Another good exercise: Stand with your arms at a 90-degree angle. Rotate them outward as you squeeze your shoulder blades together. Hold for 5 seconds and return to the starting position.

## Prevent It

- **Recondition your neck and shoulders.** Properly conditioned muscles in your neck and shoulders can help keep everything strong and supple. Your regular upper-body workout should include lots of overhead shoulder work, as well as the resistance exercises mentioned in Fix It that specifically target your neck. I also recommend yoga and Pilates for overall kinetic chain conditioning.

- **Watch your posture.** Most people spend hours each day in an office chair, and lousy posture can contribute to neck problems. While sitting, imagine a straight line from your ears down to your hips. Your shoulders should be back and open, feeling as if they're resting on your shoulder blades. This keeps your body aligned and also promotes good breathing. Also, get up, move around, and stretch at least once an hour.

## When to Call a Doctor

Muscular neck pain doesn't usually require a doctor visit. In most cases, pain resolves with conservative care within 1 to 4 weeks, depending on the severity of the problem. But if your pain doesn't respond to any home-based care within a couple of weeks, schedule an appointment with a sports doctor to see if there are any other issues to address. Your doctor may suggest other conservative measures that could help, such as acupuncture. Also, if you have a desk job, consider consulting a physical therapist about ergonomic adjustments you can make to your office chair and desk that could help.

## Do You Need Surgery?

No.

# Nerve-Based Neck Pain (Cervical Radiculopathy)

## The Symptoms

Sharp pain radiating into the shoulder and sometimes into the arm and hands, especially when lifting and/or turning your head. Variations can include numbness, tingling, or weakness.

## What's Going On in There?

Cervical radiculopathy is impossible to say three times fast, but it is more common than you think and causes a lot of confusion in athletes. This condition brings pain in the shoulder and/or arm, and athletes think something is wrong with either one or both when the problem is neither. The issue is in the neck.

Your cervical spine (the upper portion) houses your spinal cord, which has cervical nerve roots branching off to supply motor and sensory function to your upper arms. When you raise your head and/or twist your neck, the cervical nerve roots can be pinched where they exit the cervical spine. Voilà, you have pain in the shoulder or arm nerves down the line from the source.

This is called referred pain, or pain that comes from a part of the body where you don't feel it. Statistically, the most common origin point for referred pain into the upper extremities is the neck, and the most common destination for referred pain is the shoulder or arms. I see this a lot, especially in cyclists

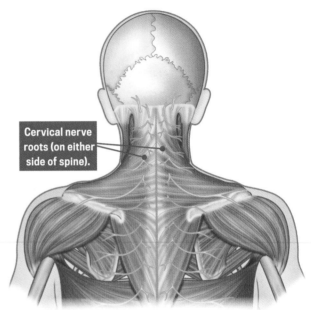

Cervical nerve roots (on either side of spine).

who have pain when they're riding in the "aero" position, bent down on their bike with their heads raised. Swimmers are also susceptible.

So what causes the problem? Your neck vertebrae may be out of alignment or you could have a degenerative issue like arthritis or bone spurs, but the most common cause in young-to-middle-aged athletes is a herniated cervical disc compressing the nerves.

## Fix It

- **See a doctor.** It's smart to see a doctor for this radiating arm or shoulder pain because a proper diagnosis usually requires some detective work. See When to Call a Doctor.

■ **Employ dynamic rest.** Avoid any activities that engage the neck and shoulders. Use lower-body workouts to maintain fitness.

■ **Ice it.** Apply ice to the neck for 15 minutes four to six times a day for the first 48 hours.

■ **Try an NSAID.** Anti-inflammatories like ibuprofen and naproxen can help with swelling and inflammation.

■ **Reestablish range of motion.** As pain improves, try these exercises to help recondition your neck and shoulders. Once you're pain free, move on to more aggressive neck and shoulder conditioning to help prevent the problem from recurring.

  ● *Neck stretches:* Stand with your hands behind your neck. Bend your neck back and look at the ceiling. Squeeze your shoulder blades together. Hold for a second and return to the starting position. Work up to 10 reps. Also try basic head rotation, left and right, as well as tilting your head to the side, left and right, for up to 10 reps each.

  ● *Basic resistance:* Do the same movements as in the above stretches, but change them to resistance exercises by using your hands to prevent your head from moving; i.e., put your hand on the right side of your head and try to tilt your head to the right while your hand prevents it. Hold for 5 seconds. Do this for left and right tilt, left and right head turn, and forward and backward movements.

  ● *Shoulder rehab:* Shoulder shrugs, holding at the top for 5 seconds, are effective. Another good exercise: Stand with your arms at a 90-degree angle. Rotate them outward as you squeeze your shoulder blades together. Hold for 5 seconds and return to the starting position.

## Prevent It

■ **Recondition your neck and shoulders.** Properly conditioned muscles in your neck and shoulders can help keep everything in its place. The stronger and more flexible the muscles, the more support your spine has, which can prevent nerve compression. Your regular upper-body workout should include lots of overhead shoulder work, as well as the resistance exercises mentioned in Fix It that specifically target your neck. I also recommend yoga and Pilates for overall kinetic chain conditioning.

■ **Watch your posture.** Most people spend hours each day in an office chair, and lousy posture can contribute to neck problems. While sitting, imagine a straight line from your ears down to your hips. Your shoulders should be back and open, feeling as if they're resting on your shoulder blades. This keeps your body aligned and also promotes good breathing. Also, get up, move around, and stretch at least once an hour.

## When to Call a Doctor

A physical exam of the neck and upper body can help offer clues as to which movements cause the pain. X-rays of the neck can show if bones are out of alignment, and an MRI can reveal cervical disc herniation.

Over-the-counter anti-inflammatories (ibuprofen or naproxen), along with icing, are generally effective against cervical radiculopathy pain. A sports doc can also use more aggressive therapies to ease symptoms. For intense pain, a short course of oral steroids can be used, and, if pain persists, the doctor can inject corticosteroids directly into the area. Physical therapy is also a mainstay of initial treatment.

## Do You Need Surgery?

Rarely. With the basic therapies listed here, most patients are asymptomatic within 2 to 4 weeks.

THE MALADY

# Tennis Elbow

## The Symptoms

Pain on the outer side of the elbow that some-times radiates into the forearm and wrist. Pain increases when you grip things, such as someone's hand or a tool.

## What's Going On in There?

Tennis elbow is actually called *lateral epicon-dylitis*, but we'll stick with tennis elbow.

The condition is a classic overuse injury, but it can also come from asking too much of an unprepared muscle. The forearm has a series of muscles on the lateral (outer) side called the extensors. You use these muscles to straighten, raise, and lower your wrist, and they're especially engaged when you're grip-ping something (such as a tennis racket or hammer).

The tendons for these extensor muscles come together at a common point and attach on a lower protrusion of the humerus (upper-arm) bone called the *lateral epicondyle*— again, "lateral" because this is the outer side of the bone. (The inner side of the bone would be "medial.")

When these tendons become irritated or strained from any repetitive wrist motion (and/or from gripping something), you have tennis elbow. The "tennis" part nods to how common this injury is for tennis players, but really, anyone who grips and swings some-thing can be at risk.

## Fix It

- **Employ dynamic rest.** Avoid any activities that engage the elbow and forearm, which includes hard gripping of objects. Use lower-body workouts to maintain fitness.

- **Ice it, then heat it.** Apply ice to the area for 15 minutes four to six times a day for the first 48 hours. After that, applying heat in the same intervals can help promote blood-flow to the tendon, which is crucial to healing.

- **Try an NSAID.** Anti-inflammatories like ibuprofen and naproxen can help with swelling and inflammation.

- **Try a strap.** A tennis elbow strap or brace can help stabilize the tendons in the elbow and keep the condition from getting worse (or prevent it in the first place).

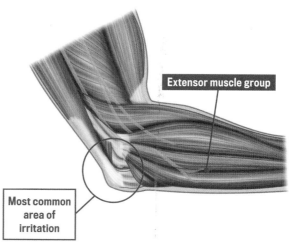

Extensor muscle group

Most common area of irritation

- **Recondition your forearm.** As pain improves, you can do some simple exercises to rehab your arm and get yourself back to normal activities. Here are three.
  - *Tennis ball squeeze:* Hold a tennis ball in your hand and squeeze for several seconds, then release. Start with a few reps and increase as pain allows. If you feel pain, back off.
  - *Arm rotations:* Hold your arm at a 90-degree angle, palm up. Make a fist. Turn your fist over as if you're flipping a pancake. Add reps as pain allows. As you get stronger, add weight to your fist, like a light dumbbell or hammer and, eventually, a racket.
  - *Wrist extension and flexion:* Do simple wrist extensions and flexions. *Extension:* With your arm bent at 90 degrees and your palm down, bend your hand back at the wrist. Hold for several seconds. Return to the starting position and repeat. *Flexion:* With your arm bent at 90 degrees and your palm up, lift your hand toward your body. Hold for several seconds. Return to the starting position and repeat. You can also add light dumbbells to these exercises as you get stronger.

## Prevent It

- **Train for your sport.** If you play a "gripping" sport that requires you to swing a racket, bat, or club or engage in any other sport or activity that requires a strong grip, you have to condition your arms, especially your forearms. The stronger and more supple your extensors, the less stress you put on the tendons and elbow. Target your forearms as part of a sport-specific training program.

- **Perfect your form.** Tennis elbow commonly results from lousy form, especially on the backhand. If tennis elbow is a problem for you, consult with a coach to evaluate and adjust your form. A bonus: Your game will probably improve!

- **Strap it.** Tennis elbow straps and braces can help prevent injury. Give one a try.

## When to Call a Doctor

Generally, tennis elbow isn't something you need a doctor for. However, more severe or persistent cases should be checked out. If your pain doesn't improve with home-based remedies in a week or two, see a sports doctor. It could be a more severe case of tennis elbow, or you could have other underlying issues. A doctor can send you for x-rays and/or an MRI to see what the trouble is.

Physical therapy is a good option here. Your doctor can also use corticosteroid injections, though that treatment is falling out of favor because—while it helps in the short term—in the long term, the pain can return, and having multiple injections can cause the tendons in the joint to deteriorate.

Platelet-rich plasma (PRP) therapy has also been shown to be effective, though it may not be covered by insurance.

## Do You Need Surgery?

Doubtful. Only in severe cases that don't respond to conservative care over months or sometimes even as long as a year would surgery become an option. A vast percentage of cases simply heal on their own.

# PART FOUR

# The Workouts

**A**nd here they are! This section gives you 40 workouts, broken out across specific benefits like total-body fitness, core strength, lower-body strength, and so on. You'll also learn how the 10-, 20-, and 30-minute sessions break down, how to tailor them to your fitness level, and how to use them to get maximum benefit. It's time to crank some tunes, fire yourself up, get sweaty, and have some fun!

# HOW A 30-MINUTE WORKOUT BREAKS DOWN

**S**tart with a minute. The foundation of the 30-minute workout lies in each individual minute, as you'll perform an interval of an exercise for 1 minute and then move on to the next exercise. How long you perform that exercise within that 1 minute time frame is up to you, and that's how the workouts can be tailored to anyone at any fitness level. You can do the exercise for 45 seconds and rest for 15. Or you can do it for 15 seconds and rest for 45. Heck, maybe starting out you can do only 5-55. That's totally cool. Everyone is different, and we all have our own levels to strive for. When you're in that minute, it's all about you—and how much you can do without breaking form. You can also tailor that work ratio as you move through the 30-minute workout: Maybe you can do 45-15 when you start, but you have to slowly dial it back to 15-45 by the time you finish. It's that simple.

**Each 30-minute workout is broken into three 10-minute segments.** There are several reasons for this.

- It allows you to adjust for your fitness level. Beginners may want (or be able) to work for only 10 or 20 minutes. That's

fine! That's how you make and measure progress. I guarantee that if you can do only 10 minutes of a workout the first week, after a few weeks you'll be doing more. Keep going!

- It allows you to ramp up, if that's your style. Some people like to pace themselves early on and then really kick it up for the last 10 minutes. It's up to you.

- It allows for a variety of exercises. Every 10 minutes you get a new set.

- It allows the exercises to become more challenging with each new set. I don't go crazy on you, but the last 10 minutes of each workout should test you harder than the first 10.

- It allows for a 1-minute rest between 10-minute sets. (You'll want it!)

**Take it 10 minutes at a time.**

- The **First 10:** Start with a 3-minute Dynamic Warmup (you'll learn what that is in a moment). Rest for 1 minute. Then perform three exercises for 1 minute each,

121

working through the set twice (that's 6 minutes, rounding out the First 10).

■ Rest for 1 minute, then begin the **Second 10**. You'll have three new exercises, perform each for 1 minute, and work through the set three times (that's 9 minutes).

■ Rest for 1 minute, then begin the **Third 10**. You'll have three new exercises, perform each for 1 minute, and work through the set three times (that's 9 minutes).

And you're done!

## WHAT EQUIPMENT DO YOU NEED?

The 30-minute workouts are designed for almost no equipment. You certainly don't need a gym membership. I want these workouts to require little to no preparation, to be portable (for the most part), and to be adaptable to your lifestyle and living space—all of which make them more difficult to skip. So here's what you need.

■ **A pair of dumbbells:** The weight will vary depending on your fitness level and what exercise you're performing, but in general, 6 to 8 pounds for women and 10 to 15 pounds for men will be plenty for most exercises. For some exercises, like the Farmer's Walk, you'll want heavier weight. Just remember that if you're experimenting, it's best to start with a low weight and have to increase rather than the other way around.

■ **A bench, box, step, or chair:** These items are interchangeable, as they function as a base for certain exercises. Steps work well because you can't beat the immovable stability, and just about everyone can find a couple of steps somewhere.

■ **And that's it!** Understand, there are lots of terrific pieces of fitness equipment out there that I could recommend: exercise bands, suspension trainers, Swiss balls, medicine balls, the BOSU ball, and even something as simple as a jump rope. If you love 'em, use 'em! But as I said, I wanted to create workouts that minimize excuses ("I couldn't get to the gym," "I don't have a TRX," etc.) and maximize convenience.

## Hey, Where Are the Pullups?

Pullups (or chinups, depending on which grip you use) are among the most simple and effective upper-body exercises. The only problem? They require a pullup bar. Just about every gym has one, and you can improvise with playground equipment and tree limbs, but the simple fact is that most people don't have instant access to a pullup bar (and probably don't want to install one at home). I designed the 30-minute workouts for convenience and simplicity. If you have a pullup bar you can use—and you want to use it—by all means sub in pullups for other upper-body exercises in the workouts. But if you don't? Not a problem. Just don't accuse me of ignoring one of the best upper-body moves ever!

# A Note for Beginners

If you're just starting out, I envy you. You're opening up a new world for yourself, and that's exciting. But workouts do require effort, and I want your experience to be positive. So remember a few things as you get moving.

- *Go slow.* Exercises are about quality of movement, not quantity. I want you performing each one with good form and deliberate motions. That's how you'll get better.

- *Accept help.* From walls, furniture, and floors, that is. If you need to use any of those things to help balance or support you as you work, by all means do so. You'll get better as you go, but I don't want you deciding not to work out because it's too difficult or intimidating. You will get the hang of it.

- *Understand the difference between soreness and pain.* General soreness is to be expected after any strength training. But pain—usually acute and localized to one area—may signal injury (a pulled hamstring, for example). See Chapter 9 for more info on injuries. An injury is rarely the end of your workout streak—it just means you have to tweak your plan. My main goal is to keep you moving!

- *Savor the gains.* When you're just starting out, you'll see quick gains. Enjoy them! Build on them. Use them as motivational fire to keep going.

## HOW TO USE THE 30-MINUTE WORKOUTS

The 30-minute workouts, as a program, are fluid. You can use them, well, pretty much any way you like. They can be your one-stop fitness solution. Or maybe you want to add one in every once in a while to break up other activities you do. Maybe you want to use them, as I do, to build muscle to enhance your performance or reach specific fitness goals (better marathon and triathlon performance for me). The workouts will serve you well in all those scenarios. But I do have a couple of suggestions.

- **Strive for an overall balance.** If these workouts are your primary fitness activity, go after them with a mind for total-body fitness. Many of the workouts are designed for your entire body, but maybe you want to give your lower body some extra work.

Excellent. But my advice is to avoid concentrating on one thing long term at the expense of another. Remember your kinetic chain.

- **Don't overdo it.** You could do a 30-minute workout three times a week and be very happy with the results. Me, I recommend some kind of physical activity 7 days a week, but I sure don't recommend 7 straight days of strength training. Being good to your body means challenging it but also respecting its need to recover and working it in ways that keep it healthy while improving it.

## YOU CAN HIIT ANYTHING

The illustrated workouts you're about to see consist of resistance (or strength-training) exercises performed at high-intensity intervals, with the intervals adjustable for any fitness level. What if on a given day, however, you don't want to strength-train and still want a HIIT workout?

That's easy: You can make any workout a HIIT session. All you have to do is use intervals instead of steady-state training. You can do that with running, cycling, swimming, jumping rope, and even walking.

You can also be creative about how you break up the intervals. Some ideas:

- Use landmarks like telephone poles or that parked car up ahead as your interval triggers.

- Use a song on your headphones (sprint for the guitar solo!).

- If you're on a treadmill with a TV screen, use the commercial breaks.

Name an exercise and you can HIIT it.

### WHAT IS A DYNAMIC WARMUP?

Before each workout, you'll perform a Dynamic Warmup for 3 minutes—six exercises, 30 seconds each. Then you'll rest for a minute and start the main workout. The

## Run Like a Little Kid

In these workouts, occasionally you'll see High Knees or The Runner or Shuttle Run finishing up a workout. Doing High Knees is an indoor solution to a potential lack of running room. That's why I recommend taking the 30-minute workouts outdoors whenever you can. One, being outside is invigorating. And two, you have room to move.

And here's something adults forget: There are no rules for movement. You can run in a circle or a figure 8 (the tighter the figure, the more challenging the sprint), slalom through a row of trees, anything. From a grown-up standpoint, changing direction and speed challenges your body in interesting ways. But from a little kid's standpoint? It just makes it more fun.

reason? A Dynamic Warmup is designed to prepare your body for the work ahead. You're pumping blood, warming up your muscles and connective tissue, and sending game-on signals to your brain. In this case, *dynamic* simply means "movement"—the exercises are very basic and designed to get you in motion, ready to sweat, and a little bit out of breath.

## But I Hate (Insert Least Favorite Exercise Here)!

You just might encounter an exercise in these workouts that you, well, don't like. Or feel strongly opposed to. Or despise.

Before you banish it from your life forever, think about why you hate it so much. Chances are—and I've gone

through this myself—the exercise is really challenging. It makes you work hard. Maybe it makes you work muscles you haven't worked before, which is where the challenge comes from—which means you probably need it more than some exercises that you enjoy

because they don't put you to such a test.

My advice: If you hate an exercise because it's hard—because it challenges you—then accept the challenge. I'll bet that after a couple of weeks, you might not hate it as much.

You've probably heard the comparison that a cold muscle is like a frozen rubber band—pull it too hard and it'll snap. But the Dynamic Warmup isn't just about preventing injury (though that is important to a guy like me). It's also about getting the most out of the workout ahead. You see, if a muscle is ready for the job it's asked to do, it will do the job more powerfully and more efficiently and, in the end, allow you to perform better overall.

You want to be at your best when you work out. The Dynamic Warmup helps get you there. You'll see the Dynamic Warmup referenced at the beginning of each exercise. Just refer back to this page to see the exercises (after a couple of sessions, you'll have them memorized).

And here they are! Perform each for 30 seconds before you begin your regular workout.

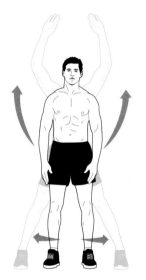

## JUMPING JACKS

Stand with your feet together and your hands at your sides. Simultaneously raise your extended arms above your head and jump up just enough to spread your feet out wide. Without pausing, quickly reverse the movement and repeat. Keep your ankles locked by pulling your toes up, and bounce on the balls of your feet.

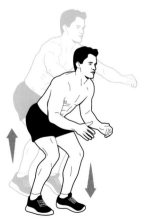

## POGO HOP

Stand in an athletic stance with your feet hip-width apart and your arms bent around 90 degrees. Keeping your body upright, repeatedly jump up, allowing only your feet to move a few inches from the floor. Keep your ankles locked, toes flexed up, and floor contact on the balls of your feet.

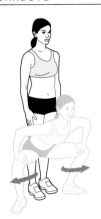

## GATE SWING

Stand with your feet together and your hands at your sides. Drop into a squat by pushing your hips back and lowering your body toward the floor, while keeping your back upright. As you lower yourself, hop your feet wider with your toes pointing outward, and gently press your hands on your inner thighs to open your knees as far as you can to facilitate the stretch. Hop back up to the starting position and repeat.

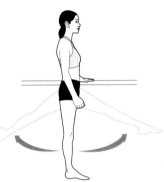

## HIP SWING

Stand tall and hold on to a sturdy object with your left hand. Brace your core. Keep your left knee straight, and swing your left leg forward as high as you comfortably can. Then, swing it backward as far as you can. That's 1 rep. Swing back and forth continuously. Complete all your reps, then do the same with your other leg.

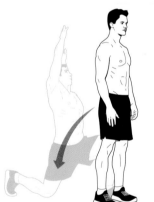

## REVERSE LUNGE AND REACHBACK

Stand tall with your feet hip-width apart. Step backward with your right leg, and lower your body until your left knee is bent at least 90 degrees. Once in this position, reach your arms up and back toward your left shoulder. Press back up to a standing position, and then step back with your left leg, this time reaching toward your right.

## INCHWORM

Stand tall with your legs straight. Bend over and touch the floor. Keeping your legs straight, walk your hands forward as far as you can without letting your hips sag. Then take tiny steps to walk your feet to your hands. That's 1 repetition.

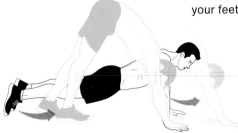

# TOTAL-BODY BASIC

These 10 workouts are designed to do just what they say: hit as many muscles as possible in the simplest way possible. Many of the exercises involve multiple muscle groups and are based on functional movement; i.e., they'll train you for natural movements you do every day. Don't be fooled by the word *basic*. You'll be familiar with some of the exercises, but these workouts will challenge anybody.

# Total-Body Basic #1

## FIRST 10

**3 MINUTES:** Do the Dynamic Warmup (page 125).

**1 MINUTE:** Rest.

**6 MINUTES:** Perform each exercise for 1 minute, cycling through the set two times.

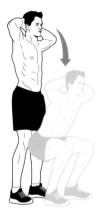

### BODYWEIGHT SQUAT

Stand with your hands on the back of your head and your feet shoulder-width apart. Lower your body until your thighs are parallel to the floor. Pause, then return to the starting position. Repeat for the allotted time.

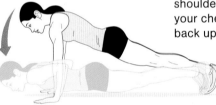

### PUSHUP

Get down on all fours, placing your hands slightly wider than your shoulders. Straighten your arms and legs. Lower your body until your chest nearly touches the floor. Pause, then push yourself back up. Repeat for the allotted time.

### PLANK

Assume a pushup position but with your weight on your forearms. Brace your abs, clench your glutes, and keep your body straight from head to heels.

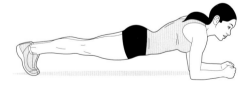

## SECOND 10

**1 MINUTE:** Rest.

**9 MINUTES:** Perform each exercise for 1 minute, cycling through the set three times.

### HIGH KNEES

(NOTE: If you have room, such as if you are working outdoors, substitute regular running sprints.) Sprint in place, bringing your knees up to your chest. Keep your back straight as you pump your arms and drive your hands past your hips in time with your legs for the allotted time.

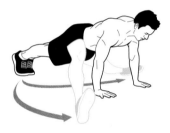

### THREE-POINT CORE TOUCH

Assume a pushup position. Quickly move your right leg forward so your right heel lands outside your right hand. Pause and return to the pushup position. Now quickly move your right leg forward so your right foot lands outside your left hand, and then return to the pushup position. That's 1 rep. Work for half the allotted time, then repeat with your left leg.

### CHANGEUP PUSHUP

Assume a pushup position with your hands close together. Do a pushup. Next place your hands shoulder-width apart. Do a pushup. Now spread your hands twice shoulder-width apart and do a pushup. Continue back to the close-hands position, and repeat the cycle for the allotted time.

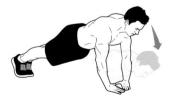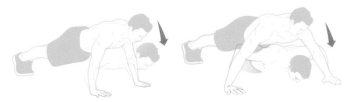

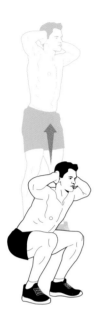

## THIRD 10

**1 MINUTE:** Rest.

**9 MINUTES:** Perform each exercise for 1 minute, cycling through the set three times.

### JUMP SQUAT

Stand with your hands on the back of your head and your feet shoulder-width apart. Lower your body until your thighs are parallel to the floor, and then jump as high as you can. When you land, immediately squat and jump again.

### ELEVATED BIRD DOG

Assume a pushup position and "walk" your feet forward so your knees are bent about 90 degrees and slightly above the floor. Raise your right arm and left leg until they're in line with your body. Return to the starting position, and then repeat with your left arm and right leg. Alternate arms and legs with each rep.

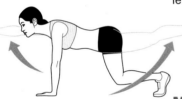

### MOUNTAIN CLIMBER

Assume a pushup position. Your body should form a straight line from your head to your ankles. Without allowing your lower-back posture to change, lift your right foot off the floor and move your right knee toward your chest. Return to the starting position, and repeat with your left leg. Alternate legs, moving quickly.

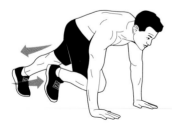

# Total-Body Basic #2

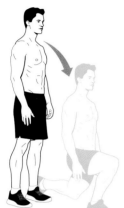

**3 MINUTES:** Do the Dynamic Warmup (page 125).

**1 MINUTE:** Rest.

**6 MINUTES:** Perform each exercise for 1 minute, cycling through the set two times.

### LUNGE

Stand with your feet hip-width apart. Step forward with your right leg and lower your body until the top of your right thigh is parallel to the floor and your left knee comes close to the floor. Pause, then return to the starting position. Alternate legs for the allotted time.

### PUSHUP

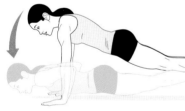

Get down on all fours, placing your hands slightly wider than your shoulders. Straighten your arms and legs. Lower your body until your chest nearly touches the floor. Pause, then push yourself back up. Repeat for the allotted time.

### BICYCLE CRUNCH

Lie faceup with your hips and knees bent 90 degrees so that your lower legs are parallel to the floor. Clasp your hands behind your head. Lift your shoulders off the floor and hold them there. Twist your upper body to the right as you bring your right knee in as fast as you can until it touches your left elbow. Simultaneously straighten your left leg. Return to the starting position and repeat to the other side.

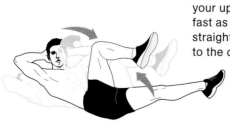

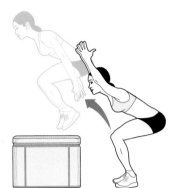

## SECOND 10

**1 MINUTE:** Rest.

**9 MINUTES:** Perform each exercise for 1 minute, cycling through the set three times.

### BOX JUMP

Stand in front of a knee-high box, bench, or step with your arms raised. Drive your arms down, dip your knees, and jump onto the box. Step down.

### DUMBBELL STRAIGHT-LEG DEADLIFT AND ROW

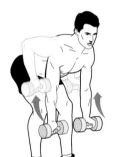

Stand with your knees slightly bent and hold a pair of dumbbells at arm's length in front of your thighs. Without rounding your lower back or changing the bend in your knees, bend at your hips and lower your torso until it's nearly parallel to the floor. Without moving your torso, pull the dumbbells up to the sides of your chest. Pause, then lower the dumbbells. Raise your torso back to the starting position.

### BENCH DIP

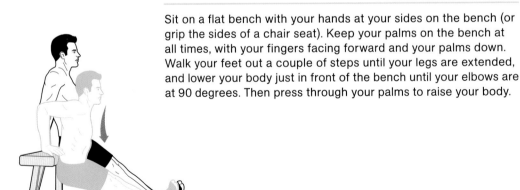

Sit on a flat bench with your hands at your sides on the bench (or grip the sides of a chair seat). Keep your palms on the bench at all times, with your fingers facing forward and your palms down. Walk your feet out a couple of steps until your legs are extended, and lower your body just in front of the bench until your elbows are at 90 degrees. Then press through your palms to raise your body.

## THIRD 10

**1 MINUTE:** Rest.

**9 MINUTES:** Perform each exercise for 1 minute, cycling through the set three times.

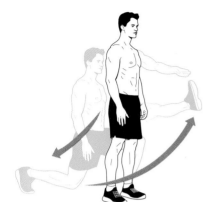

### REVERSE LUNGE WITH TOE TOUCH

Stand with your feet hip-width apart. Step back with your right leg and lower your body until your knee almost touches the floor. Stand up, swing your right leg as high as you can, and touch your toes with your left hand. Alternate sides for the allotted time.

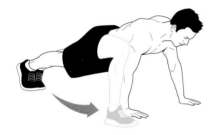

### LIZARD CRAWL

Position your body on the floor in a pushup position. Walk forward with your left arm as you simultaneously lift your right foot up and step forward. With each step, you should lower your body toward the floor. Continue this alternating action, like you are crawling but with your knees off the floor. With each step of your foot, your knee will come close to touching your elbow. Your back should stay straight throughout the range of motion.

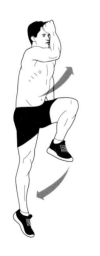

### HIGH KNEES

(NOTE: If you have room, such as if you are working outdoors, substitute regular running sprints.) Sprint in place, bringing your knees up to your chest. Keep your back straight as you pump your arms and drive your hands past your hips in time with your legs for the allotted time.

# Total-Body Basic #3

## FIRST 10

**3 MINUTES:** Do the Dynamic Warmup (page 125).

**1 MINUTE:** Rest.

**6 MINUTES:** Perform each exercise for 1 minute, cycling through the set two times.

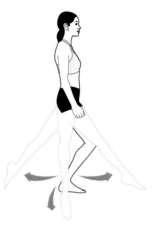

### THREE-POINT BALANCE TOUCH

Standing on your left leg with your knee slightly bent and chest up, perform a quarter squat. Your right leg (the nonbalancing leg) will perform the following three actions while the rest of your body remains still.

A. Reach your right foot as far forward as possible and gently tap the floor, then return to the starting position.

B. Next reach your right foot out to the right as far as possible, tap the floor with your toes, and return to the starting position.

C. Finally, reach your right foot as far back behind you as possible, touch the floor with your toes, and return to the starting position.

That's 1 repetition. Alternate legs for the allotted time. The deeper you squat, the harder this exercise becomes.

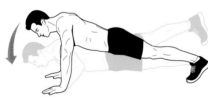

### SINGLE-LEG PUSHUP

Assume a pushup position. While descending, lift your right leg 8 to 10 inches off the floor. Return to the starting position and descend again, this time raising your left leg. Alternate for the allotted time.

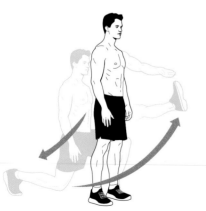

### REVERSE LUNGE WITH TOE TOUCH

Stand with your feet hip-width apart. Step back with your right leg and lower your body until your knee almost touches the floor. Stand up, swing your right leg as high as you can, and touch your toes with your left hand. Alternate sides for the allotted time.

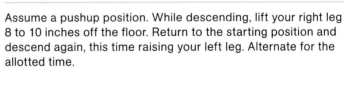

## SECOND 10

**1 MINUTE:** Rest.

**9 MINUTES:** Perform each exercise for 1 minute, cycling through the set three times.

## BURPEE WITH PUSHUP

Stand with your feet shoulder-width apart. Squat as deeply as you can and place your hands on the floor. Kick back into a pushup position. Do 1 pushup. Bring your legs back to a squat and jump up. Land and repeat.

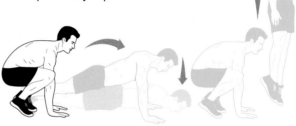

## DUMBBELL ROW

Holding a dumbbell in each hand, bend at your hips and knees and lower your torso until it's nearly parallel to the floor. Let the dumbbells hang at arm's length. Now pull the dumbbells up to the sides of your chest. Pause, then slowly lower them.

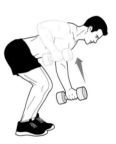

## THE RUNNER

Lie on your back with your legs straight, elbows at your sides, and arms bent 90 degrees. This is the starting position. Lift your shoulders and back off the floor as you bring your left knee toward your chest and drive your right arm forward (as if you're running). Return to the starting position. Repeat with your right knee and left arm and alternate sides.

## THIRD 10

**1 MINUTE:** Rest.

**9 MINUTES:** Perform each exercise for 1 minute, cycling through the set three times.

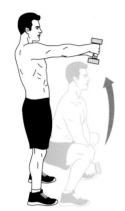

### DUMBBELL SWING

(NOTE: You can also use a kettlebell for this exercise.) Using both hands, hold a dumbbell by one end with your arms hanging straight down in front of you. Stand with your feet hip-width apart, chest up, and shoulders back. Bend your knees slightly and push the weight back between your legs, then explode forward and upward with your hips to propel the weight out in front of you. Brace your core and squeeze your glutes as you swing the weight up, using momentum, until the weight is at chest height. In a smooth motion, swing the weight back down between your legs. Repeat.

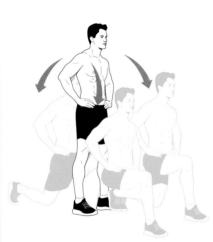

### COMPASS LUNGE

Stand with your feet hip-width apart. Step forward (or "north") with your right leg and lower your body until the top of your right thigh is parallel to the floor and your left knee comes close to the floor. Push back to standing and repeat the exercise while hitting points on the compass (northeast, east, etc.). (NOTE: Northern lunges are forward; southern are reverse; east and west are side lunges.) When you hit "due south," switch legs and continue until you reach north again. Do as much as you can in the allotted time.

### SINGLE-LEG, SINGLE-ARM PLANK

Assume a pushup position but with your weight on your forearms. Brace your abs, clench your glutes, and keep your body straight from head to heels. Raise your left leg and extend your right arm out in front of you. Hold for 5 seconds, then lower your arm and leg and raise your right leg/left arm for 5 seconds. Alternate for the allotted time.

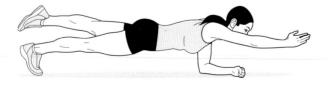

# Total-Body Basic #4

**3 MINUTES:** Do the Dynamic Warmup (page 125).

**1 MINUTE:** Rest.

**6 MINUTES:** Perform each exercise for 1 minute, cycling through the set two times.

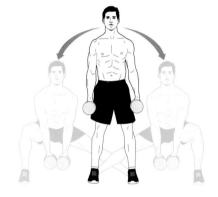

## LOW SIDE-TO-SIDE LUNGE

Stand with your feet shoulder-width apart and clasp your hands in front of your chest (or hold dumbbells, as illustrated). Shift your weight to your right leg and lower your body, bending your right knee and pushing your butt back. Keep your left leg straight and left foot flat on the floor. Without raising yourself all the way to standing, shift the movement to the left. Alternate back and forth. (NOTE: Be sure to push your hips back as you lower down and engage your core to keep your upper body vertical.)

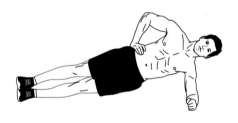

## SIDE PLANK

Lie on your left side, prop yourself up on your left forearm, and raise your hips so your body is straight from ankles to head. Hold for half the allotted time, then switch sides and repeat.

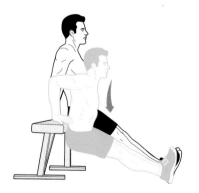

## BENCH DIP

Sit on a flat bench with your hands at your sides on the bench (or grip the sides of a chair seat). Keep your palms on the bench at all times, with your fingers facing forward and your palms down. Walk your feet out a couple of steps until your legs are extended, and lower your body just in front of the bench until your elbows are at 90 degrees. Then press through your palms to raise your body.

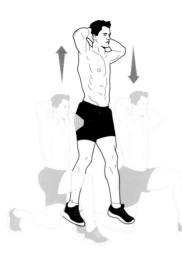

## SECOND 10

**1 MINUTE:** Rest.

**9 MINUTES:** Perform each exercise for 1 minute, cycling through the set three times.

### BODYWEIGHT SPLIT JUMP

Place your hands behind your head and assume a staggered stance, right leg forward. Slowly lower your body as far as you can, then jump with enough force to propel both feet off the floor. Land with your left leg forward. That's 1 rep. Alternate back and forth for the allotted time.

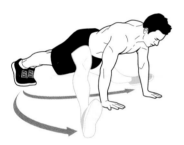

### THREE-POINT CORE TOUCH

Assume a pushup position. Quickly move your right leg forward so your right heel lands outside your right hand. Pause and return to the pushup position. Now quickly move your right leg forward so your right foot lands outside your left hand, and then return to the pushup position. That's 1 rep. Work for half the allotted time, then repeat with your left leg.

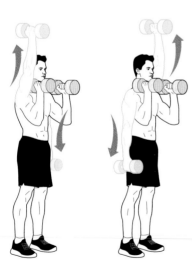

### ALTERNATING DUMBBELL CURL AND PRESS

Stand with a pair of dumbbells just outside your shoulders, arms bent, and palms facing each other. Press the right dumbbell overhead as you lower the left one to your side. Reverse the move as you return to the starting position, then press the left dumbbell overhead and lower the right. Alternate for the allotted time.

## THIRD 10

**1 MINUTE:** Rest.

**9 MINUTES:** Perform each exercise for 1 minute, cycling through the set three times.

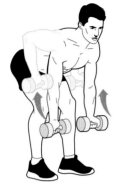

### DUMBBELL STRAIGHT-LEG DEADLIFT AND ROW

Stand with your knees slightly bent and hold a pair of dumbbells at arm's length in front of your thighs. Without rounding your lower back or changing the bend in your knees, bend at your hips and lower your torso until it's nearly parallel to the floor. Without moving your torso, pull the dumbbells up to the sides of your chest. Pause, then lower the dumbbells. Raise your torso back to the starting position.

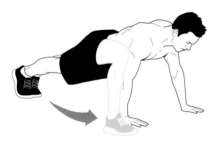

### LIZARD CRAWL

Position your body on the floor in a pushup position. Walk forward with your left arm as you simultaneously lift your right foot up and step forward. With each step, you should lower your body toward the floor. Continue this alternating action, like you are crawling but with your knees off the floor. With each step of your foot, your knee will come close to touching your elbow. Your back should stay straight throughout the range of motion.

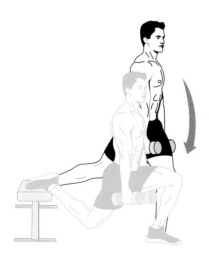

### DUMBBELL BULGARIAN SPLIT SQUAT

Hold a pair of dumbbells at arm's length next to your hips. Stand in a staggered stance and place the top of your back foot on a bench, step, or chair. Keeping your torso upright, bend your front knee and lower your body as far as you can. Pause, then push back to the starting position. Halfway through the allotted time, switch legs.

# Total-Body Basic #5

**FIRST 10**

**3 MINUTES:** Do the Dynamic Warmup (page 125).

**1 MINUTE:** Rest.

**6 MINUTES:** Perform each exercise for 1 minute, cycling through the set two times.

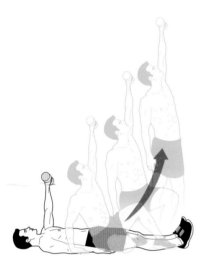

## TURKISH GET-UP

Lie on your back with your right arm by your side and a dumbbell or kettlebell in your left hand above your chest. Now roll onto your right side, prop up on your right forearm, and push yourself into a half kneel by threading your right leg behind your left. Stand up to complete the move. Reverse it to return to the starting position. Switch sides halfway through the allotted time.

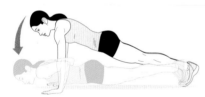

## PUSHUP

Get down on all fours, placing your hands slightly wider than your shoulders. Straighten your arms and legs. Lower your body until your chest nearly touches the floor. Pause, then push yourself back up. Repeat for the allotted time.

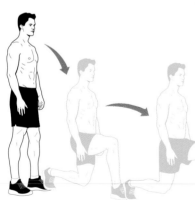

## WALKING LUNGE (FORWARD AND REVERSE)

Stand with your feet hip-width apart. Step forward with your right leg and lower your body until the top of your right thigh is parallel to the floor and your left knee comes close to the floor. Without rising, lunge forward with your left leg. Keep your torso upright and swing your arms in a running motion with each lunge. Alternate legs for half the allotted time, then perform reverse lunges back to the starting point.

## SECOND 10

**1 MINUTE:** Rest.

**9 MINUTES:** Perform each exercise for 1 minute, cycling through the set three times.

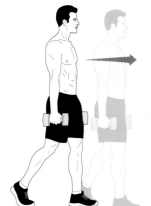

### FARMER'S WALK

Grab a pair of heavy dumbbells and let them hang naturally at arm's length by your sides, holding them as tightly as possible. Now walk for as long as you can before your grip starts to fail. (Walk forward and backward for equal amounts of time; for an added challenge, walk on your toes to target your calves.) If you can walk for longer than 1 minute, try heavier weights.

### MOUNTAIN CLIMBER

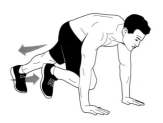

Assume a pushup position. Your body should form a straight line from your head to your ankles. Without allowing your lower-back posture to change, lift your right foot off the floor and move your right knee toward your chest. Return to the starting position, and repeat with your left leg. Alternate legs, moving quickly.

### HIP-UP

Lie on your left side, your right arm extended so it's perpendicular to the floor. Prop yourself up on your left forearm and raise your hips so your body is straight from ankles to head. Lower your left hip, and then raise it again until it's in line with your body. Halfway through the allotted time, switch sides and repeat.

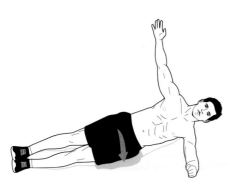

## THIRD 10

**1 MINUTE:** Rest.

**9 MINUTES:** Perform each exercise for 1 minute, cycling through the set three times.

### SUMO BURPEE

Stand with your feet several inches wider than your shoulders, then squat (like a sumo wrestler) and place your hands on the floor in front of you. Kick your legs back into a pushup position, quickly bring your legs back to a squat, and jump up, throwing your hands above your head. Land and repeat.

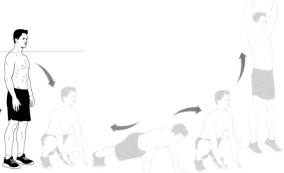

### DUMBBELL HAMMER CURL AND PRESS

Standing with your feet shoulder-width apart, hold a pair of dumbbells at arm's length by your sides, palms facing each other. Without moving your upper arms, curl the weights to your shoulders, then press them overhead until your arms are straight. Reverse the move to return to the starting position.

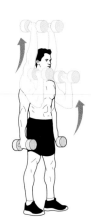

### CRAB ROLL

Sit, knees bent, with your palms and feet on the floor. Raise your hips so your body is in a straight line from your knees to your shoulders; this is the starting position. Lift your right foot and left hand and flip over to your right, placing your left hand back on the floor and kicking your right leg out behind you. (Keep it elevated.) Flip back to the starting position. That's 1 rep.

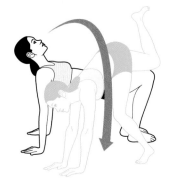

# Total-Body Basic #6

**3 MINUTES:** Do the Dynamic Warmup (page 125).

**1 MINUTE:** Rest.

**6 MINUTES:** Perform each exercise for 1 minute, cycling through the set two times.

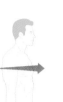

### FARMER'S WALK

Grab a pair of heavy dumbbells and let them hang naturally at arm's length by your sides, holding them as tightly as possible. Now walk for as long as you can before your grip starts to fail. (Walk forward and backward for equal amounts of time; for an added challenge, walk on your toes to target your calves.) If you can walk for longer than 1 minute, try heavier weights.

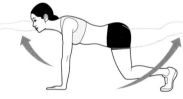

### ELEVATED BIRD DOG

Assume a pushup position and "walk" your feet forward so your knees are bent about 90 degrees and slightly above the floor. Raise your right arm and left leg until they're in line with your body. Return to the starting position, and then repeat with your left arm and right leg. Alternate arms and legs with each rep.

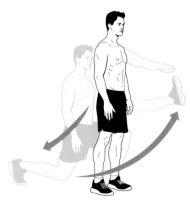

### REVERSE LUNGE WITH TOE TOUCH

Stand with your feet hip-width apart. Step back with your right leg and lower your body until your knee almost touches the floor. Stand up, swing your right leg as high as you can, and touch your toes with your left hand. Alternate sides for the allotted time.

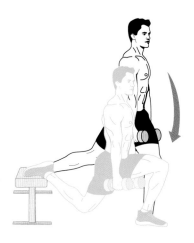

**SECOND 10**

**1 MINUTE:** Rest.

**9 MINUTES:** Perform each exercise for 1 minute, cycling through the set three times.

## DUMBBELL BULGARIAN SPLIT SQUAT

Hold a pair of dumbbells at arm's length next to your hips. Stand in a staggered stance and place the top of your back foot on a bench, step, or chair. Keeping your torso upright, bend your front knee and lower your body as far as you can. Pause, then push back to the starting position. Halfway through the allotted time, switch legs.

## LIZARD CRAWL

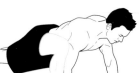

Position your body on the floor in a pushup position. Walk forward with your left arm as you simultaneously lift your right foot up and step forward. With each step, you should lower your body toward the floor. Continue this alternating action, like you are crawling but with your knees off the floor. With each step of your foot, your knee will come close to touching your elbow. Your back should stay straight throughout the range of motion.

## BENCH DIP

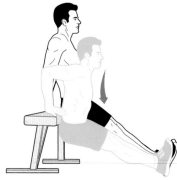

Sit on a flat bench with your hands at your sides on the bench (or grip the sides of a chair seat). Keep your palms on the bench at all times, with your fingers facing forward and your palms down. Walk your feet out a couple of steps until your legs are extended, and lower your body just in front of the bench until your elbows are at 90 degrees. Then press through your palms to raise your body.

## THIRD 10

**1 MINUTE:** Rest.

**9 MINUTES:** Perform each exercise for 1 minute, cycling through the set three times.

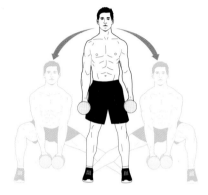

### LOW SIDE-TO-SIDE LUNGE

Stand with your feet shoulder-width apart and clasp your hands in front of your chest (or hold dumbbells, as illustrated). Shift your weight to your right leg and lower your body, bending your right knee and pushing your butt back. Keep your left leg straight and left foot flat on the floor. Without raising yourself all the way to standing, shift the movement to the left. Alternate back and forth. (NOTE: Be sure to push your hips back as you lower down and engage your core to keep your upper body vertical.)

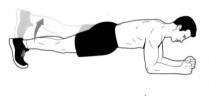

### SINGLE-LEG PLANK

Assume a pushup position but with your weight on your forearms. Brace your abs, clench your glutes, and keep your body straight from head to heels. Raise your right leg and hold it for 5 seconds. Then lower it and raise your left leg for 5 seconds. Alternate legs for the allotted time.

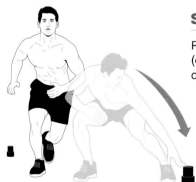

### SHUTTLE RUN

Place two cones or other kinds of markers 10 to 25 yards apart (depending on how much room you have). Sprint from one to the other and back.

# Total-Body Basic #7

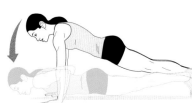

**3 MINUTES:** Do the Dynamic Warmup (page 125).

**1 MINUTE:** Rest.

**6 MINUTES:** Perform each exercise for 1 minute, cycling through the set two times.

## PUSHUP

Get down on all fours, placing your hands slightly wider than your shoulders. Straighten your arms and legs. Lower your body until your chest nearly touches the floor. Pause, then push yourself back up. Repeat for the allotted time.

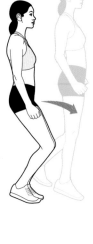

## MULTIDIRECTIONAL HOP

Stand with your knees slightly bent. Jump forward 12 inches and land on your right foot. Hop backward to the starting position, landing on both feet. Repeat on your left foot. Next do the sequence going sideways. Continue throughout the allotted time. (Hold a dumbbell in front of your chest with both hands for an added challenge.)

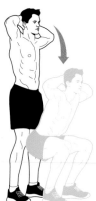

## BODYWEIGHT SQUAT

Stand with your hands on the back of your head and your feet shoulder-width apart. Lower your body until your thighs are parallel to the floor. Pause, then return to the starting position. Repeat for the allotted time.

## SECOND 10

**1 MINUTE:** Rest.

**9 MINUTES:** Perform each exercise for 1 minute, cycling through the set three times.

### INCHWORM

Stand tall with your legs straight. Bend over and touch the floor. Keeping your legs straight, walk your hands forward as far as you can without letting your hips sag. Then take tiny steps to walk your feet to your hands. That's 1 repetition.

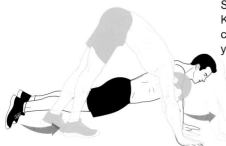

### MOGUL JUMP

Get on all fours and lift your knees a few inches off the floor so your weight is on your hands and the balls of your feet. Keeping your arms straight and legs together, hop, rotating your knees and feet to the right. Now hop as you rotate your knees and feet to the left. That's 1 rep. Alternate sides for the allotted time.

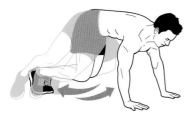

### SIDE PLANK

Lie on your left side, prop yourself up on your left forearm, and raise your hips so your body is straight from ankles to head. Hold for half the allotted time, then switch sides and repeat.

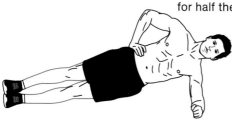

## THIRD 10

**1 MINUTE:** Rest.

**9 MINUTES:** Perform each exercise for 1 minute, cycling through the set three times.

### CLOSE-HANDS PUSHUP

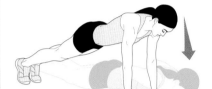

Assume a pushup position with your hands about 6 inches apart (your body should form a straight line from your ankles to your head). Brace your abs, squeeze your glutes, and keep your elbows tucked in against your sides as you lower yourself until your chest is about an inch from the floor. Pause, then push up to the starting position.

### LEG TUCK AND TWIST

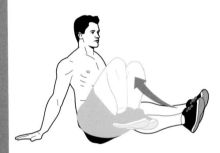

Sit on the floor, leaning back 45 degrees, your legs straight and palms on the floor behind you. Lift your legs off the floor. Pull your knees toward your left shoulder as you twist your torso to your left. Return to the starting position and repeat to your right.

### HIGH KNEES

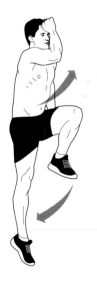

(NOTE: If you have room, such as if you are working outdoors, substitute regular running sprints.) Sprint in place, bringing your knees up to your chest. Keep your back straight as you pump your arms and drive your hands past your hips in time with your legs for the allotted time.

# Total-Body Basic #8

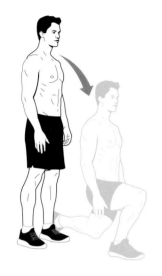

**3 MINUTES:** Do the Dynamic Warmup (page 125).

**1 MINUTE:** Rest.

**6 MINUTES:** Perform each exercise for 1 minute, cycling through the set two times.

### LUNGE

Stand with your feet hip-width apart. Step forward with your right leg and lower your body until the top of your right thigh is parallel to the floor and your left knee comes close to the floor. Pause, then return to the starting position. Alternate legs for the allotted time.

### PLANK

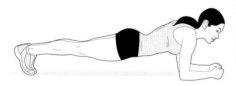

Assume a pushup position but with your weight on your forearms. Brace your abs, clench your glutes, and keep your body straight from head to heel.

### CHANGEUP PUSHUP

Assume a pushup position with your hands close together. Do a pushup. Next place your hands shoulder-width apart. Do a pushup. Now spread your hands twice shoulder-width apart and do a pushup. Continue back to the close-hands position, and repeat the cycle for the allotted time.

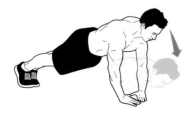 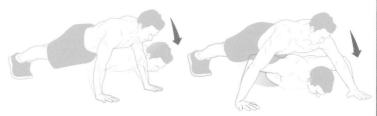

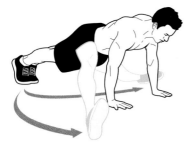

## SECOND 10

**1 MINUTE:** Rest.

**9 MINUTES:** Perform each exercise for 1 minute, cycling through the set three times.

## THREE-POINT CORE TOUCH

Assume a pushup position. Quickly move your right leg forward so your right heel lands outside your right hand. Pause and return to the pushup position. Now quickly move your right leg forward so your right foot lands outside your left hand, and then return to the pushup position. That's 1 rep. Work for half the allotted time, then repeat with your left leg.

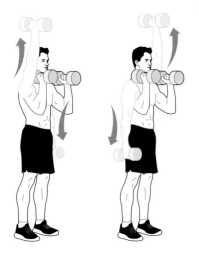

## ALTERNATING DUMBBELL CURL AND PRESS

Stand with a pair of dumbbells just outside your shoulders, arms bent, and palms facing each other. Press the right dumbbell overhead as you lower the left one to your side. Reverse the move as you return to the starting position, then press the left dumbbell overhead and lower the right. Alternate for the allotted time.

## DUMBBELL STRAIGHT-LEG DEADLIFT

Hold a pair of dumbbells in front of your thighs with your feet hip-width apart and your knees slightly bent. Hinge forward at your hips, lowering your torso until it's nearly parallel to the floor. Pause, then return to the starting position.

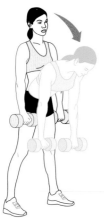

## THIRD 10

**1 MINUTE:** Rest.

**9 MINUTES:** Perform each exercise for 1 minute, cycling through the set three times.

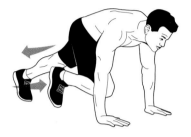

### MOUNTAIN CLIMBER

Assume a pushup position. Your body should form a straight line from your head to your ankles. Without allowing your lower-back posture to change, lift your right foot off the floor and move your right knee toward your chest. Return to the starting position, and repeat with your left leg. Alternate legs, moving quickly.

### SINGLE-LEG HIP RAISE

Lie on your back with your left knee bent and left foot flat on the floor. Raise your right leg so it's in line with your left thigh. Push your hips up, keeping your right leg elevated. Pause, then slowly return to the starting position. Switch legs halfway through the allotted time.

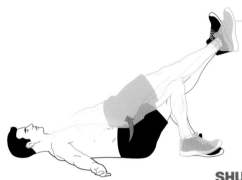

### SHUTTLE RUN

Place two cones or other kinds of markers 10 to 25 yards apart (depending on how much room you have). Sprint from one to the other and back.

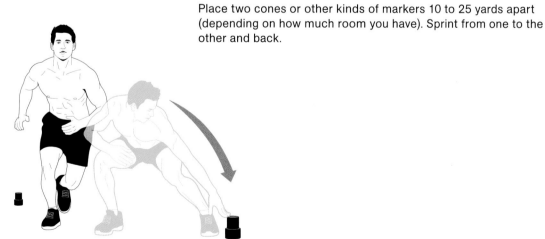

# Total-Body Basic #9

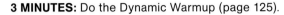

**3 MINUTES:** Do the Dynamic Warmup (page 125).

**1 MINUTE:** Rest.

**6 MINUTES:** Perform each exercise for 1 minute, cycling through the set two times.

## SQUAT JUMP

Stand with your feet shoulder-width apart and hands on hips. Now squat with your heels flat and touch the floor with your palms. Jump forcefully, thrusting your arms overhead with palms inward to boost your momentum. Land and immediately begin the next jump.

## PRONE COBRA

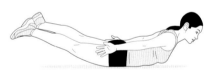

Lie facedown on the floor with your legs straight and your arms at your sides, palms down. Contract your glutes and lift your head, chest, arms, and legs off the floor. Simultaneously rotate your arms so your thumbs point toward the ceiling. Your hips should be the only part of your body touching the floor. Hold for a 5 count, then return to the starting position. Perform as many reps as you can in the allotted time.

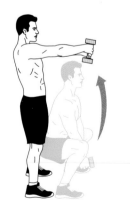

## DUMBBELL SWING

(NOTE: You can also use a kettlebell for this exercise.) Using both hands, hold a dumbbell by one end with your arms hanging straight down in front of you. Stand with your feet hip-width apart, chest up, and shoulders back. Bend your knees slightly and push the weight back between your legs, then explode forward and upward with your hips to propel the weight out in front of you. Brace your core and squeeze your glutes as you swing the weight up, using momentum, until the weight is at chest height. In a smooth motion, swing the weight back down between your legs. Repeat.

## SECOND 10

**1 MINUTE:** Rest.

**9 MINUTES:** Perform each exercise for 1 minute, cycling through the set three times.

### REVERSE PUSHUP

Assume a pushup position with your arms straight and hands slightly wider than your shoulders. Bend at the elbows and lower your torso until your chest nearly touches the floor. Pause, then push your butt toward your ankles until your knees are bent 90 degrees. Return to the starting position and repeat.

### THE RUNNER

Lie on your back with your legs straight, elbows at your sides, and arms bent 90 degrees. This is the starting position. Lift your shoulders and back off the floor as you bring your left knee toward your chest and drive your right arm forward (as if you're running). Return to the starting position. Repeat with your right knee and left arm and alternate sides.

### SUMO BURPEE

Stand with your feet several inches wider than your shoulders, then squat (like a sumo wrestler) and place your hands on the floor in front of you. Kick your legs back into a pushup position, quickly bring your legs back to a squat, and jump up, throwing your hands above your head. Land and repeat.

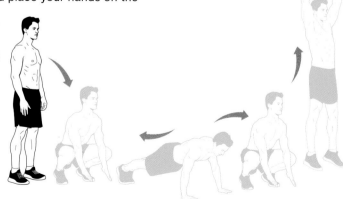

## THIRD 10

**1 MINUTE:** Rest.

**9 MINUTES:** Perform each exercise for 1 minute, cycling through the set three times.

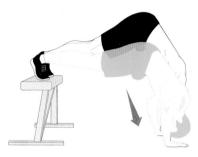

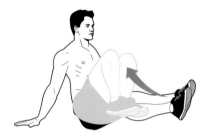

### INVERTED SHOULDER PRESS

Assume a pushup position with your feet on a bench or chair. Push your hips up so your torso is nearly perpendicular to the floor. Your hands should be slightly wider than your shoulders and your arms straight. Without changing your body posture, lower yourself until your head nearly touches the floor. Pause, then return to the starting position.

### LEG TUCK AND TWIST

Sit and lean back 45 degrees, your legs straight and palms on the floor behind you. Lift your legs off the floor. Pull your knees toward your left shoulder as you twist your torso to your left. Return to the starting position and repeat to your right.

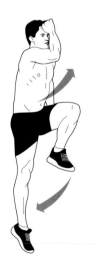

### HIGH KNEES

(NOTE: If you have room, such as working outdoors, substitute regular running sprints.) Sprint in place, bringing your knees up to your chest. Keep your back straight as you pump your arms and drive your hands past your hips in time with your legs. Alternate knees for the allotted time.

# Total-Body Basic #10

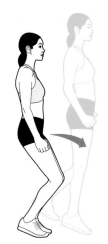

## FIRST 10

**3 MINUTES:** Do the Dynamic Warmup (page 125).

**1 MINUTE:** Rest.

**6 MINUTES:** Perform each exercise for 1 minute, cycling through the set two times.

### MULTIDIRECTIONAL HOP

Stand with your knees slightly bent. Jump forward 12 inches and land on your right foot. Hop backward to the start, landing on both feet. Repeat on your left foot. Next, do the sequence going sideways. Continue throughout the allotted time. (Hold a dumbbell in front of your chest with both hands for an added challenge.)

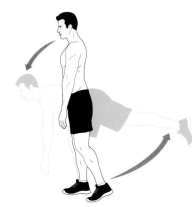

### SINGLE-LEG, STRAIGHT-LEG DEADLIFT REACH

Stand with your arms at your sides. Raise your left foot and left hand. Slowly lower your torso and touch the toes of your right foot with your left hand. Return to the starting position. Work for half the allotted time and switch sides.

### INVERTED SHOULDER PRESS

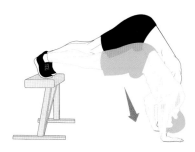

Assume the pushup position with your feet on a bench or chair. Push your hips up so your torso is nearly perpendicular to the floor. Your hands should be slightly wider than your shoulders and your arms straight. Without changing your body posture, lower yourself until your head nearly touches the floor. Pause, then return to the starting position.

## SECOND 10

**1 MINUTE:** Rest.

**9 MINUTES:** Perform each exercise for 1 minute, cycling through the set three times.

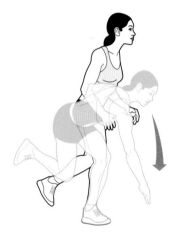

### SKATER HOP

This exercise mimics the explosive side-to-side movements of speed skaters. Stand on your right foot with your right knee slightly bent, and place your left foot back behind your right ankle. Bend your right knee and lower your body into a partial squat. Then explosively bound to the left by jumping off your right foot. Land on your left foot and bring your right foot back behind your left foot. Reach your right hand toward your left foot. Hop back to the right, landing on your right foot and reaching for the floor with your left hand (touch the floor if you're able). Repeat, alternating sides.

### HIP RAISE

Lie faceup on the floor with your knees bent and your feet flat on the floor. Raise your hips so your body forms a straight line from your shoulders to your knees. Clench your glutes as you reach the top of the movement. Pause, then lower your body back to the starting position.

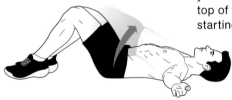

### PLANK

Assume a pushup position but with your weight on your forearms. Brace your abs, clench your glutes, and keep your body straight from head to heels.

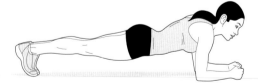

## THIRD 10

**1 MINUTE:** Rest.

**9 MINUTES:** Perform each exercise for 1 minute, cycling through the set three times.

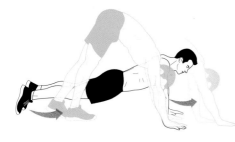

### INCHWORM

Stand tall with your legs straight. Bend over and touch the floor. Keeping your legs straight, walk your hands forward as far as you can without letting your hips sag. Then take tiny steps to walk your feet to your hands. That's 1 repetition.

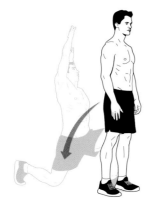

### REVERSE LUNGE AND REACHBACK

Stand tall with your feet hip-width apart. Step backward with your right leg, and lower your body until your left knee is bent at least 90 degrees. Once in this position, reach your arms up and back toward your left shoulder. Press back up to a standing position, and then step back with your left leg, this time reaching toward your right.

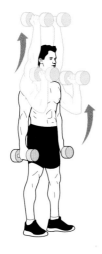

### DUMBBELL HAMMER CURL AND PRESS

Standing with your feet shoulder-width apart, hold a pair of dumbbells at arm's length by your sides, palms facing each other. Without moving your upper arms, curl the weights to your shoulders, then press them overhead until your arms are straight. Reverse the move to return to the starting position.

# PLYO EXPLOSION

These workouts will put a spring in your step. The exercises add an element of plyometric explosiveness— enough that you'll spend a good portion of the workouts airborne. The key to these sessions is smoothness and control. Maintain good form so you keep your balance during takeoffs and landings. You want strong glutes, not a bruised butt.

# Plyo Explosion #1

**3 MINUTES:** Do the Dynamic Warmup (page 125).

**1 MINUTE:** Rest.

**6 MINUTES:** Perform each exercise for 1 minute, cycling through the set two times.

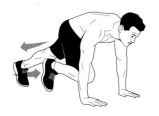

### MOUNTAIN CLIMBER

Assume a pushup position. Your body should form a straight line from your head to your ankles. Without allowing your lower-back posture to change, lift your right foot off the floor and move your right knee toward your chest. Return to the starting position, and repeat with your left leg. Alternate legs, moving quickly.

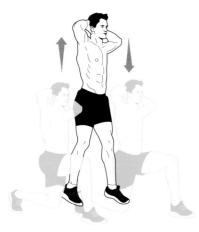

### BODYWEIGHT SPLIT JUMP

Place your hands behind your head and assume a staggered stance, right leg forward. Slowly lower your body as far as you can, then jump with enough force to propel both feet off the floor. Land with your left leg forward. That's 1 rep. Alternate back and forth for the allotted time.

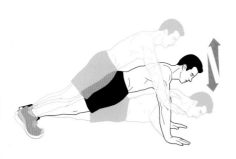

### PLYO PUSHUP

Assume a pushup position, with your hands slightly beyond shoulder width and your body in a straight line from head to ankles. Bend your elbows and lower your body until your chest nearly touches the floor, then push up with enough force that your hands leave the floor. (NOTE: Control your motion to soften the landing on your wrists to prevent injury.) To make this exercise easier, elevate your hands on a step, bench, or box.

**1 MINUTE:** Rest.

**9 MINUTES:** Perform each exercise for 1 minute, cycling through the set three times.

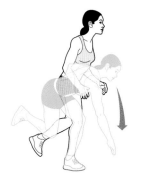

## SKATER HOP

This exercise mimics the explosive side-to-side movements of speed skaters. Stand on your right foot with your right knee slightly bent, and place your left foot back behind your right ankle. Bend your right knee and lower your body into a partial squat. Then explosively bound to the left by jumping off your right foot. Land on your left foot and bring your right foot back behind your left foot. Reach your right hand toward your left foot. Hop back to the right, landing on your right foot and reaching for the floor with your left hand (try to touch the floor). Repeat, alternating sides.

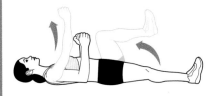

## THE RUNNER

Lie on your back with your legs straight, elbows at your sides, and arms bent 90 degrees. This is the starting position. Lift your shoulders and back off the floor as you bring your left knee toward your chest and drive your right arm forward (as if you're running). Return to the starting position. Repeat with your right knee and left arm and alternate sides.

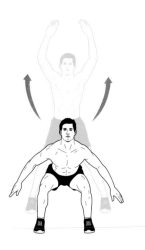

## STAR JUMP

With your feet about shoulder-width apart, squat down so your hands move down to the floor near your feet. Then, in one movement, jump up into the air and spread your arms and legs out as wide as you possibly can. Return to the starting position and repeat.

## THIRD 10

**1 MINUTE:** Rest.

**9 MINUTES:** Perform each exercise for 1 minute, cycling through the set three times.

## DUMBBELL SWING

(NOTE: You can also use a kettlebell for this exercise.) Using both hands, hold a dumbbell by one end with your arms hanging straight down in front of you. Stand with your feet hip-width apart, chest up, and shoulders back. Bend your knees slightly and push the weight back between your legs, then explode forward and upward with your hips to propel the weight out in front of you. Brace your core and squeeze your glutes as you swing the weight up, using momentum, until the weight is at chest height. In a smooth motion, swing the weight back down between your legs. Repeat.

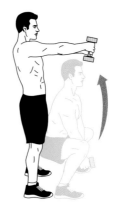

## HIGH KNEES

(NOTE: If you have room, such as if you are working outdoors, substitute regular running sprints.) Sprint in place, bringing your knees up to your chest. Keep your back straight as you pump your arms and drive your hands past your hips in time with your legs for the allotted time.

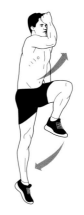

## "DEATH CRAWL" WITH DUMBBELL JUMP SQUAT

Assume a pushup position, grasping a dumbbell in each hand. Do a pushup, then row the dumbbell in your right hand up to the side of your chest and lower it to the floor. Do the same with your left arm. Now "walk" the dumbbell in your left hand forward one step, followed by the one in your right. Next bring your left foot, then right foot, forward. Move ahead three steps with each hand. Keep your core tense and back straight throughout the movement. Then stand up and do 3 dumbbell jump squats (holding the dumbbells at your sides, bend your knees and squat, then jump up explosively). That's 1 rep. Alternate walking forward and backward. Do as much as you can in the allotted time.

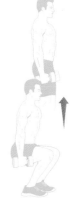

# Plyo Explosion #2

## FIRST 10

**3 MINUTES:** Do the Dynamic Warmup (page 125).

**1 MINUTE:** Rest.

**6 MINUTES:** Perform each exercise for 1 minute, cycling through the set two times.

### MULTIDIRECTIONAL HOP

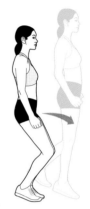

Stand with your knees slightly bent. Jump forward 12 inches and land on your right foot. Hop backward to the starting position, landing on both feet. Repeat on your left foot. Next do the sequence going sideways. Continue for the allotted time. (Hold a dumbbell in front of your chest with both hands for an added challenge.)

### BURPEE WITH PUSHUP

Stand with your feet shoulder-width apart. Squat as deeply as you can and place your hands on the floor. Kick back into a pushup position. Do 1 pushup. Bring your legs back to a squat and jump up. Land and repeat. (NOTE: For a bigger challenge, perform a Plyo Pushup—see page 159.)

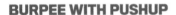

### BICYCLE CRUNCH

Lie faceup with your hips and knees bent 90 degrees so that your lower legs are parallel to the floor. Clasp your hands behind your head. Lift your shoulders off the floor and hold them there. Twist your upper body to the right as you bring your right knee in as fast as you can until it touches your left elbow. Simultaneously straighten your left leg. Return to the starting position and repeat to the other side.

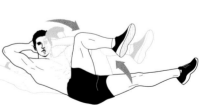

**SECOND 10**

**1 MINUTE:** Rest.

**9 MINUTES:** Perform each exercise for 1 minute, cycling through the set three times.

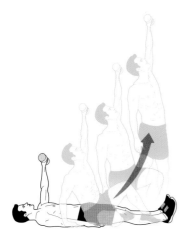

### TURKISH GET-UP

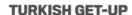

Lie on your back with your right arm by your side and a dumbbell or kettlebell in your left hand above your chest. Now roll onto your right side, prop up on your right forearm, and push yourself into a half kneel by threading your right leg behind your left. Stand up to complete the move. Reverse it to return to the starting position. Switch sides halfway through your time.

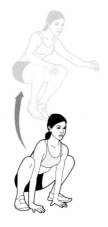

### FROG JUMP

Squat and touch the floor with both hands, keeping your arms straight. Then explode into the air, raising your knees as high as they'll go. Land and immediately begin the next jump.

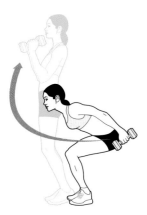

### DUMBBELL SKIER SWING

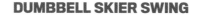

Holding a pair of dumbbells at arm's length next to your sides, stand with your knees slightly bent. Without rounding your lower back, bend at your hips as you simultaneously swing your arms backward. Now explosively thrust your hips forward and raise your torso until you're standing upright, while allowing your momentum to swing the weights up to chest level. (Don't actively lift the weights.) Swing back and forth for the allotted time.

**THIRD 10**

**1 MINUTE:** Rest.

**9 MINUTES:** Perform each exercise for 1 minute, cycling through the set three times.

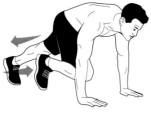

## MOUNTAIN CLIMBER

Assume a pushup position. Your body should form a straight line from your head to your ankles. Without allowing your lower-back posture to change, lift your right foot off the floor and move your right knee toward your chest. Return to the starting position, and repeat with your left leg. Alternate legs, moving quickly.

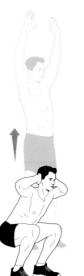

## SQUAT JUMP

Stand with your feet shoulder-width apart and hands on hips. Now squat with your heels flat and touch the floor with your palms. Jump forcefully, thrusting your arms overhead with palms inward to boost your momentum. Land and immediately begin the next jump.

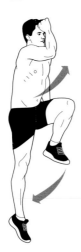

## HIGH KNEES

(NOTE: If you have room, such as if you are working outdoors, substitute regular running sprints.) Sprint in place, bringing your knees up to your chest. Keep your back straight as you pump your arms and drive your hands past your hips in time with your legs for the allotted time.

# Plyo Explosion #3

**3 MINUTES:** Do the Dynamic Warmup (page 125).

**1 MINUTE:** Rest.

**6 MINUTES:** Perform each exercise for 1 minute, cycling through the set two times.

## BOX JUMP

Stand in front of a knee-high box, bench, or step with your arms raised. Drive your arms down, dip your knees, and jump onto the box. Step down.

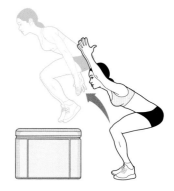

## CRAB ROLL

Sit, knees bent, with your palms and feet on the floor. Raise your hips so your body is in a straight line from your knees to your shoulders; this is the starting position. Lift your left foot and right hand and flip over to your left, placing your right hand back on the floor and kicking your left leg out behind you. (Keep it elevated.) Flip back to the starting position. That's 1 rep.

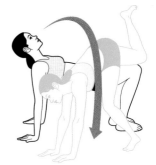

## BURPEE WITH PUSHUP

Stand with your feet shoulder-width apart. Squat as deeply as you can and place your hands on the floor. Kick back into a pushup position. Do 1 pushup. Bring your legs back to a squat and jump up. Land and repeat.

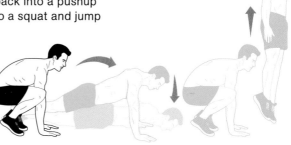

## SECOND 10

**1 MINUTE:** Rest.

**9 MINUTES:** Perform each exercise for 1 minute, cycling through the set three times.

### MOGUL JUMP

Get on all fours and lift your knees a few inches off the floor so your weight is on your hands and the balls of your feet. Keeping your arms straight and legs together, hop, rotating your knees and feet to the right. Now hop as you rotate your knees and feet to the left. That's 1 rep. Alternate sides for the allotted time.

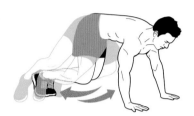

### PLYO PUSHUP

Assume a pushup position with your hands slightly beyond shoulder width and your body in a straight line from head to ankles. Bend your elbows and lower your body until your chest nearly touches the floor, then push up with enough force that your hands leave the floor. (NOTE: Control your motion to soften the landing on your wrists to prevent injury.) To make this exercise easier, elevate your hands on a step, bench, or box.

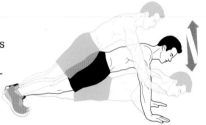

### SPLIT-JACK CURL

Hold a pair of dumbbells at your sides, palms in, feet hip-width apart. Jump into a split stance—left leg forward—while curling the weights to your shoulders. Return to the starting position and repeat, landing with your right leg forward. Alternate for the allotted time.

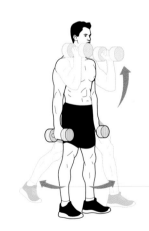

## THIRD 10

**1 MINUTE:** Rest.

**9 MINUTES:** Perform each exercise for 1 minute, cycling through the set three times.

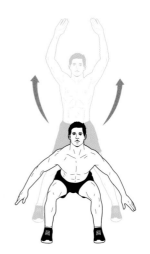

### STAR JUMP

With your feet about shoulder-width apart, squat, moving your hands down to the floor near your feet. Then, in one movement, jump up into the air and spread your arms and legs out as wide as you possibly can. Return to the starting position and repeat.

### "DEATH CRAWL" WITH DUMBBELL JUMP SQUAT

Assume a pushup position, grasping one dumbbell in each hand. Do a pushup, then row the dumbbell in your right hand up to the side of your chest and lower it to the floor. Do the same with your left arm. Now "walk" the dumbbell in your left hand forward one step, followed by the one in your right. Next bring your left foot, then right foot, forward. Move ahead three steps with each hand. Keep your core tense and back straight throughout the move-ment. Then stand up and do 3 dumbbell jump squats (holding the dumbbells at your sides, bend your knees and squat, then jump up explosively). That's 1 rep. Alternate walking forward and back-ward. Do as much as you can in the allotted time.

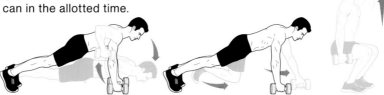

### SHUTTLE RUN

Place two cones or other kinds of markers 10 to 25 yards apart (depending on how much room you have). Sprint from one to the other and back.

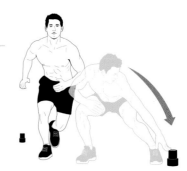

# Plyo Explosion #4

**3 MINUTES:** Do the Dynamic Warmup (page 125).

**1 MINUTE:** Rest.

**6 MINUTES:** Perform each exercise for 1 minute, cycling through the set two times.

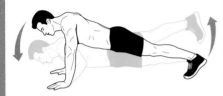

### SINGLE-LEG PUSHUP

Assume a pushup position. While descending, lift your right leg 8 to 10 inches off the floor. Return to the starting position and descend again, this time raising your left leg. Alternate for the allotted time.

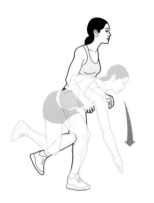

### SKATER HOP

This exercise mimics the explosive side-to-side movements of speed skaters. Stand on your right foot with your right knee slightly bent, and place your left foot back behind your right ankle. Bend your right knee and lower your body into a partial squat. Then explosively bound to the left by jumping off your right foot. Land on your left foot and bring your right foot back behind your left foot. Reach your right hand toward your left foot. Hop back to the right, landing on your right foot and reaching for the floor with your left hand (touch the floor if you're able). Repeat, alternating sides.

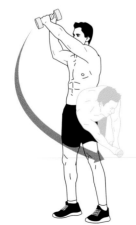

### DUMBBELL CHOP

Hold a dumbbell above your right shoulder with both hands. Stand with your feet shoulder-width apart. Brace your core and rotate your torso to the right. While keeping your arms straight, swing the dumbbell down and to the outside of your left knee by rotating to the left and bending at your hips. Reverse the movement to return to the starting position. Halfway through the prescribed time, switch sides.

## SECOND 10

**1 MINUTE:** Rest.

**9 MINUTES:** Perform each exercise for 1 minute, cycling through the set three times.

## BOX JUMP

Stand in front of a knee-high box, bench, or step with your arms raised. Drive your arms down, dip your knees, and jump onto the box. Step down.

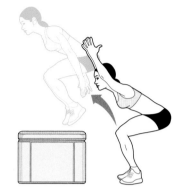

## DUMBBELL LUNGE, CURL, AND PRESS

Stand holding a pair of dumbbells at your sides, palms facing each other and feet hip-width apart. Keeping your torso upright, step forward with your left foot and lower your body until your left knee is bent 90 degrees. Hold that position and curl the dumbbells to your shoulders. Then press the dumbbells above your shoulders until your arms are straight. Lower the dumbbells back to your sides, and then push yourself back to the starting position. Alternate legs for the allotted time.

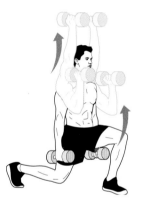

## SUMO BURPEE

Stand with your feet several inches wider than your shoulders, then squat (like a sumo wrestler) and place your hands on the floor in front of you. Kick your legs back into a pushup position, quickly bring your legs back to a squat, and jump up, throwing your hands above your head. Land and repeat.

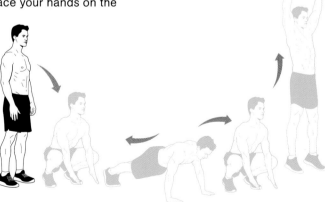

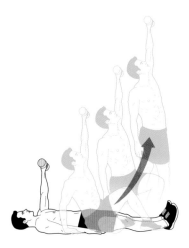

## THIRD 10

**1 MINUTE:** Rest.

**9 MINUTES:** Perform each exercise for 1 minute, cycling through the set three times.

### TURKISH GET-UP

Lie on your back with your right arm by your side and a dumbbell or kettlebell in your left hand above your chest. Now roll onto your right side, prop up on your right forearm, and push yourself into a half kneel by threading your right leg behind your left. Stand up to complete the move. Reverse it to return to the starting position. Switch sides halfway through your time.

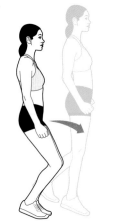

### MULTIDIRECTIONAL HOP

Stand with your knees slightly bent. Jump forward 12 inches and land on your right foot. Hop backward to the starting position, landing on both feet. Repeat on your left foot. Next do the sequence going sideways. Continue through the allotted time. (Hold a dumbbell in front of your chest with both hands for an added challenge.)

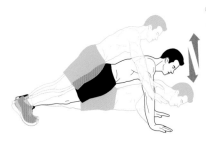

### PLYO PUSHUP

Assume a pushup position, with your hands slightly beyond shoulder width and your body in a straight line from head to ankles. Bend your elbows and lower your body until your chest nearly touches the floor, then push up with enough force that your hands leave the floor. (NOTE: Control your motion to soften the landing on your wrists to prevent injury.) To make this exercise easier, elevate your hands on a step, bench, or box.

# Plyo Explosion #5

## FIRST 10

**3 MINUTES:** Do the Dynamic Warmup (page 125).

**1 MINUTE:** Rest.

**6 MINUTES:** Perform each exercise for 1 minute, cycling through the set two times.

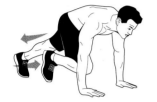

### MOUNTAIN CLIMBER

Assume a pushup position. Your body should form a straight line from your head to your ankles. Without allowing your lower-back posture to change, lift your right foot off the floor and move your right knee toward your chest. Return to the starting position, and repeat with your left leg. Alternate legs, moving quickly.

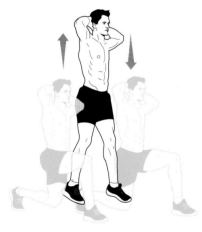

### BODYWEIGHT SPLIT JUMP

Place your hands behind your head and assume a staggered stance, right leg forward. Slowly lower your body as far as you can, then jump with enough force to propel both feet off the floor. Land with your left leg forward. That's 1 rep. Alternate back and forth for the allotted time.

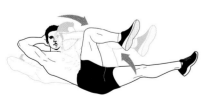

### BICYCLE CRUNCH

Lie faceup with your hips and knees bent 90 degrees so that your lower legs are parallel to the floor. Clasp your hands behind your head. Lift your shoulders off the floor and hold them there. Twist your upper body to the right as you bring your right knee in as fast as you can until it touches your left elbow. Simultaneously straighten your left leg. Return to the starting position and repeat to the other side.

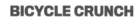

**1 MINUTE:** Rest.

**9 MINUTES:** Perform each exercise for 1 minute, cycling through the set three times.

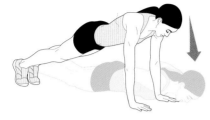

## CLOSE-HANDS PUSHUP

Assume a pushup position with your hands about 6 inches apart (your body should form a straight line from your ankles to your head). Brace your abs, squeeze your glutes, and keep your elbows tucked in against your sides as you lower yourself until your chest is about an inch from the floor. Pause, then push up to the starting position.

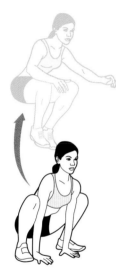

## FROG JUMP

Squat and touch the floor with both hands, keeping your arms straight. Then explode into the air, raising your knees as high as they'll go. Land and immediately begin the next jump.

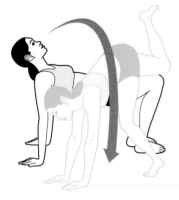

## CRAB ROLL

Sit, knees bent, with your palms and feet on the floor. Raise your hips so your body is in a straight line from your knees to your shoulders; this is the starting position. Lift your right foot and left hand and flip over to your right, placing your left hand back on the floor and kicking your right leg out behind you. (Keep it elevated.) Flip back to the starting position. That's 1 rep.

## THIRD 10

**1 MINUTE:** Rest.

**9 MINUTES:** Perform each exercise for 1 minute, cycling through the set three times.

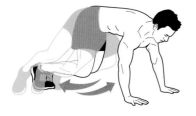

### MOGUL JUMP

Get on all fours and lift your knees a few inches off the floor so your weight is on your hands and the balls of your feet. Keeping your arms straight and legs together, hop, rotating your knees and feet to the right. Now hop as you rotate your knees and feet to the left. That's 1 rep. Alternate sides for the allotted time.

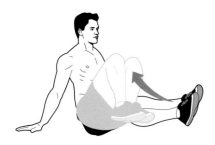

### LEG TUCK AND TWIST

Sit on the floor, leaning back 45 degrees, your legs straight and palms on the floor behind you. Lift your legs off the floor. Pull your knees toward your left shoulder as you twist your torso to your left. Return to the starting position and repeat to your right.

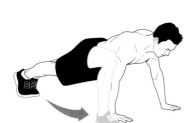

### LIZARD CRAWL

Position your body on the floor in a pushup position. Walk forward with your left arm as you simultaneously lift your right foot up and step forward. With each step, you should lower your body toward the floor. Continue this alternating action, like you are crawling but with your knees off the floor. With each step of your foot, your knee will come close to touching your elbow. Your back should stay straight throughout the range of motion.

# ANYWHERE, ANYTIME

Sometimes workouts have to do more than just make you sweat. This group does you a big favor: It eliminates excuses. These sessions require no equipment and are designed to be done in a very small area: Think bedroom, rec room, hotel room, or anywhere you have a bit of floor space. So simple! All you have to do is tie your shoes and get it done. (Heck, you don't even need shoes; try 'em barefoot!)

# Anywhere, Anytime #1

## FIRST 10

**3 MINUTES:** Do the Dynamic Warmup (page 125).

**1 MINUTE:** Rest.

**6 MINUTES:** Perform each exercise for 1 minute, cycling through the set two times.

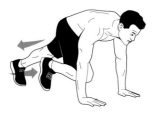

### SINGLE-LEG TOE TOUCHES

Stand on your left leg with your right leg out in front of you, raised off the floor. Extend your arms straight out at your sides at shoulder height. Bend your left leg at the knee and squat down to touch your right hand to the toe of your left foot, then come back up. Repeat with your right leg and continue, alternating for the allotted time.

### MOUNTAIN CLIMBER

Assume a pushup position. Your body should form a straight line from your head to your ankles. Without allowing your lower-back posture to change, lift your right foot off the floor and move your right knee toward your chest. Return to the starting position, and repeat with your left leg. Alternate legs, moving quickly.

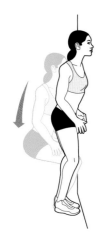

### RUSSIAN WALL SQUAT

Face a wall with your feet shoulder-width apart and toes touching the wall. Keep your arms by your sides and squat until your thighs are parallel to the floor. Pause, then return to the starting position.

## SECOND 10

**1 MINUTE:** Rest.

**9 MINUTES:** Perform each exercise for 1 minute, cycling through the set three times.

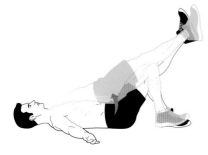

### SINGLE-LEG HIP RAISE

Lie on your back with your left knee bent and left foot flat on the floor. Raise your right leg so it's in line with your left thigh. Push your hips up, keeping your right leg elevated. Pause, then slowly return to the starting position. Switch legs halfway through the allotted time.

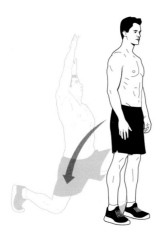

### REVERSE LUNGE AND REACHBACK

Stand tall with your feet hip-width apart. Step backward with your right leg, and lower your body until your left knee is bent at least 90 degrees. Once in this position, reach your arms up and back toward your left shoulder. Press back up to a standing position, and then step back with your left leg, this time reaching toward your right.

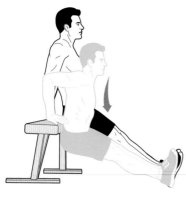

### BENCH DIP

Sit on a flat bench with your hands at your sides on the bench (or grip the sides of a chair seat). Keep your palms on the bench at all times, with your fingers facing forward and your palms down. Walk your feet out a couple of steps until your legs are extended, and lower your body just in front of the bench until your elbows are at 90 degrees. Then press through your palms to raise your body.

## THIRD 10

**1 MINUTE:** Rest.

**9 MINUTES:** Perform each exercise for 1 minute, cycling through the set three times.

### SINGLE-LEG, SINGLE-ARM PLANK

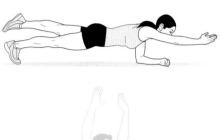

Assume a pushup position but with your weight on your forearms. Brace your abs, clench your glutes, and keep your body straight from head to heels. Raise your left leg and extend your right arm out in front of you. Hold for 5 seconds, then lower your arm and leg and raise your right leg/left arm for 5 seconds. Alternate for the allotted time.

### SQUAT JUMP

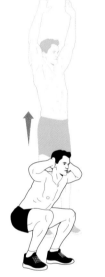

Stand with your feet shoulder-width apart and hands on hips. Now squat with your heels flat and touch the floor with your palms. Jump forcefully, thrusting your arms overhead with palms inward to boost your momentum. Land and immediately begin the next jump.

### CHANGEUP PUSHUP

Assume a pushup position with your hands close together. Do a pushup. Next place your hands shoulder-width apart. Do a pushup. Now spread your hands twice shoulder-width apart and do a pushup. Continue reps back to the close-hands position, and repeat the cycle for the allotted time.

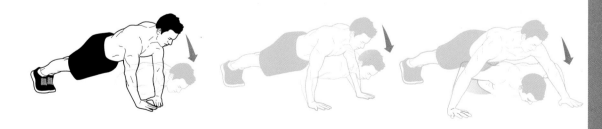

# Anywhere, Anytime #2

## FIRST 10

**3 MINUTES:** Do the Dynamic Warmup (page 125).

**1 MINUTE:** Rest.

**6 MINUTES:** Perform each exercise for 1 minute, cycling through the set two times.

### SINGLE-LEG, STRAIGHT-LEG DEADLIFT REACH

From a standing position, raise your left foot and left hand. Slowly lower your torso and touch the toes of your right foot with your left hand. Return to the starting position. Work for half the allotted time and switch sides.

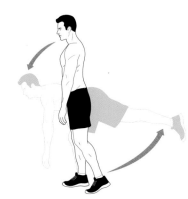

### BURPEE WITH PUSHUP

Stand with your feet shoulder-width apart. Squat as deeply as you can and place your hands on the floor. Kick back into a pushup position. Do 1 pushup. Bring your legs back to a squat and jump up. Land and repeat.

### REVERSE LUNGE WITH TOE TOUCH

Stand with your feet hip-width apart. Step back with your right leg and lower your body until your knee almost touches the floor. Stand up, swing your right leg as high as you can, and touch your toes with your left hand. Alternate sides for the allotted time.

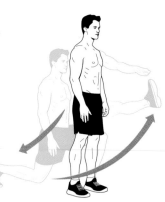

## SECOND 10

**1 MINUTE:** Rest.

**9 MINUTES:** Perform each exercise for 1 minute, cycling through the set three times.

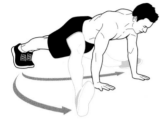

### THREE-POINT CORE TOUCH

Assume a pushup position. Quickly move your right leg forward so your right heel lands outside your right hand. Pause and return to the pushup position. Now quickly move your right leg forward so your right foot lands outside your left hand, and then return to the pushup position. That's 1 rep. Work for half the allotted time, then repeat with your left leg.

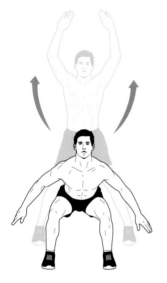

### STAR JUMP

With your feet about shoulder-width apart, squat so your hands move down to the floor near your feet. Then, in one movement, jump up into the air and spread your arms and legs out as wide as you possibly can. Return to the starting position and repeat.

### SINGLE-LEG, STRAIGHT-LEG DEADLIFT REACH

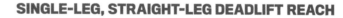

Stand with your arms at your sides. Raise your left foot and left hand. Slowly lower your torso and touch the toes of your right foot with your left hand. Return to the starting position. Work for half the allotted time and switch sides.

## THIRD 10

**1 MINUTE:** Rest.

**9 MINUTES:** Perform each exercise for 1 minute, cycling through the set three times.

### REVERSE PUSHUP

Assume a pushup position with your arms straight and hands slightly wider than your shoulders. Bend at the elbows and lower your torso until your chest nearly touches the floor. Pause, then push your butt toward your ankles until your knees are bent 90 degrees. Return to the starting position and repeat.

### SIDE PLANK

Lie on your left side, prop yourself up on your left forearm, and raise your hips so your body is straight from ankles to head. Hold for half the allotted time, then switch sides and repeat.

### BODYWEIGHT SPLIT JUMP

Place your hands behind your head and assume a staggered stance, right leg forward. Slowly lower your body as far as you can, then jump with enough force to propel both feet off the floor. Land with your left leg forward. That's 1 rep. Alternate back and forth for the allotted time.

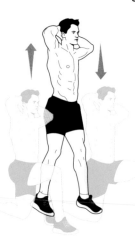

# Anywhere, Anytime #3

**3 MINUTES:** Do the Dynamic Warmup (page 125).

**1 MINUTE:** Rest.

**6 MINUTES:** Perform each exercise for 1 minute, cycling through the set two times.

## BODYWEIGHT SQUAT

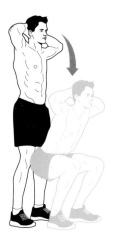

Stand with your hands on the back of your head and your feet shoulder-width apart. Lower your body until your thighs are parallel to the floor. Pause, then return to the starting position. Repeat for the allotted time.

## BICYCLE CRUNCH

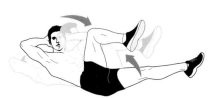

Lie faceup with your hips and knees bent 90 degrees so that your lower legs are parallel to the floor. Clasp your hands behind your head. Lift your shoulders off the floor and hold them there. Twist your upper body to the right as you bring your right knee in as fast as you can until it touches your left elbow. Simultaneously straighten your left leg. Return to the starting position and repeat to the other side.

## INCHWORM

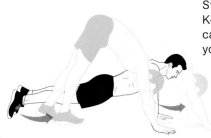

Stand tall with your legs straight. Bend over and touch the floor. Keeping your legs straight, walk your hands forward as far as you can without letting your hips sag. Then take tiny steps to walk your feet to your hands. That's 1 repetition.

## SECOND 10

**1 MINUTE:** Rest.

**9 MINUTES:** Perform each exercise for 1 minute, cycling through the set three times.

### SUMO BURPEE

Stand with your feet several inches wider than your shoulders, then squat (like a sumo wrestler) and place your hands on the floor in front of you. Kick your legs back into a pushup position, quickly bring your legs back to a squat, and jump up, throwing your hands above your head. Land and repeat.

### HIP-UP

Lie on your left side, your right arm extended so it's perpendicular to the floor. Prop yourself up on your left forearm and raise your hips so your body is straight from ankles to head. Lower your left hip, and then raise it again until it's in line with your body. Halfway through the allotted time, switch sides and repeat.

### PUSHUP

Get down on all fours, placing your hands slightly wider than your shoulders. Straighten your arms and legs. Lower your body until your chest nearly touches the floor. Pause, then push yourself back up. Repeat for the allotted time.

## THIRD 10

**1 MINUTE:** Rest.

**9 MINUTES:** Perform each exercise for 1 minute, cycling through the set three times.

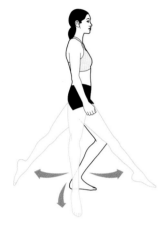

### THREE-POINT BALANCE TOUCH

Standing on your left leg with your knee slightly bent and chest up, perform a quarter squat. Your right leg (the nonbalancing leg) will perform the following three actions while the rest of your body remains still.

A. Reach your right foot as far forward as possible and gently tap the floor, then return to the starting position.

B. Next reach your right foot out to the right as far as possible, tap the floor with your toes, and return to the starting position.

C. Finally, reach your right foot as far back behind you as possible, touch the floor with your toes, and return to the starting position.

That's 1 repetition. Alternate legs for the allotted time. The deeper you squat, the harder this exercise becomes.

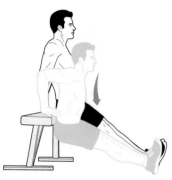

### BENCH DIP

Sit on a flat bench with your hands at your sides on the bench (or grip the sides of a chair seat). Keep your palms on the bench at all times, with your fingers facing forward and your palms down. Walk your feet out a couple of steps until your legs are extended, and lower your body just in front of the bench until your elbows are at 90 degrees. Then press through your palms to raise your body.

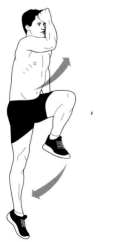

### HIGH KNEES

(NOTE: If you have room, such as if you are working outdoors, substitute regular running sprints.) Sprint in place, bringing your knees up to your chest. Keep your back straight as you pump your arms and drive your hands past your hips in time with your legs for the allotted time.

# Anywhere, Anytime #4

## FIRST 10

**3 MINUTES:** Do the Dynamic Warmup (page 125).

**1 MINUTE:** Rest.

**6 MINUTES:** Perform each exercise for 1 minute, cycling through the set two times.

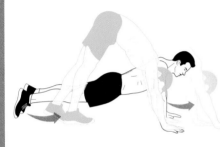

### INCHWORM

Stand tall with your legs straight. Bend over and touch the floor. Keeping your legs straight, walk your hands forward as far as you can without letting your hips sag. Then take tiny steps to walk your feet to your hands. That's 1 repetition.

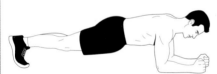

### PLANK

Assume a pushup position but with your weight on your forearms. Brace your abs, clench your glutes, and keep your body straight from head to heels.

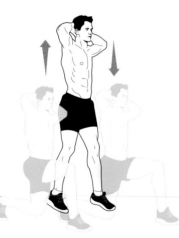

### BODYWEIGHT SPLIT JUMP

Place your hands behind your head and assume a staggered stance, right leg forward. Slowly lower your body as far as you can, then jump with enough force to propel both feet off the floor. Land with your left leg forward. That's 1 rep. Alternate back and forth for the allotted time.

## SECOND 10

**1 MINUTE:** Rest.

**9 MINUTES:** Perform each exercise for 1 minute, cycling through the set three times.

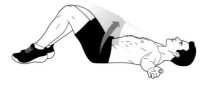

### HIP RAISE

Lie faceup on the floor with your knees bent and your feet flat on the floor. Raise your hips so your body forms a straight line from your shoulders to your knees. Clench your glutes as you reach the top of the movement. Pause, then lower your body back to the starting position.

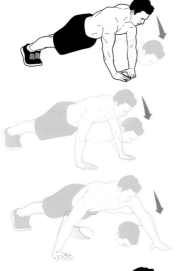

### CHANGEUP PUSHUP

Assume a pushup position with your hands close together. Do a pushup. Next place your hands shoulder-width apart. Do a pushup. Now spread your hands twice shoulder-width apart and do a pushup. Continue reps back to the close-hands position, and repeat the cycle for the allotted time.

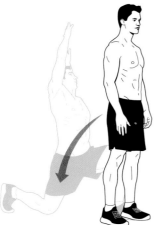

### REVERSE LUNGE AND REACHBACK

Stand tall with your feet hip-width apart. Step backward with your right leg, and lower your body until your left knee is bent at least 90 degrees. Once in this position, reach your arms up and back toward your left shoulder. Press back up to a standing position, and then step back with your left leg, this time reaching toward your right.

## THIRD 10

**1 MINUTE:** Rest.

**9 MINUTES:** Perform each exercise for 1 minute, cycling through the set three times.

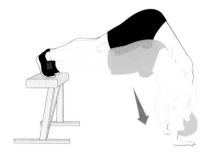

### INVERTED SHOULDER PRESS

Assume a pushup position with your feet on a bench or chair. Push your hips up so your torso is nearly perpendicular to the floor. Your hands should be slightly wider than your shoulders and your arms straight. Without changing your body posture, lower yourself until your head nearly touches the floor. Pause, then return to the starting position.

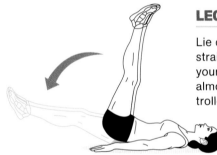

### LEGS-DOWN

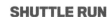

Lie on your back, legs straight and together. Keeping your legs straight, bring them all the way up and reach for the ceiling until your butt comes off the floor. Slowly lower your legs back down almost to the floor, and then raise them back up again. Use a controlled motion throughout the exercise.

### SHUTTLE RUN

Place two cones or other kinds of markers 10 to 25 yards apart (depending on how much room you have). Sprint from one to the other and back.

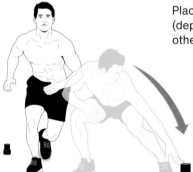

# Anywhere, Anytime #5

## FIRST 10

**3 MINUTES:** Do the Dynamic Warmup (page 125).

**1 MINUTE:** Rest.

**6 MINUTES:** Perform each exercise for 1 minute, cycling through the set two times.

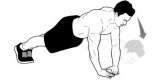

### CHANGEUP PUSHUP

Assume a pushup position with your hands close together. Do a pushup. Next place your hands shoulder-width apart. Do a pushup. Now spread your hands twice shoulder-width apart and do a pushup. Continue reps back to the close-hands position, and repeat the cycle for the allotted time.

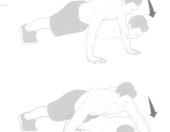

### SINGLE-LEG HIP RAISE

Lie on your back with your left knee bent and left foot flat on the floor. Raise your right leg so it's in line with your left thigh. Push your hips up, keeping your right leg elevated. Pause, then slowly return to the starting position. Switch legs halfway through the allotted time.

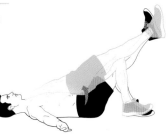

### BODYWEIGHT BULGARIAN SPLIT SQUAT

Stand in a staggered stance, your left foot 2 to 3 feet in front of your right. Place just the instep of your back foot on a bench or chair. Pull your shoulders back and brace your core. Lower your body as deeply as you can, keeping your back foot on the bench. Keep your shoulders back and chest up throughout the movement. Pause, then return to the starting position. Halfway through the prescribed time, switch feet.

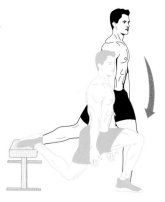

## SECOND 10

**1 MINUTE:** Rest.

**9 MINUTES:** Perform each exercise for 1 minute, cycling through the set three times.

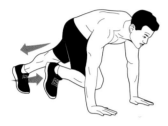

### MOUNTAIN CLIMBER

Assume a pushup position. Your body should form a straight line from your head to your ankles. Without allowing your lower-back posture to change, lift your right foot off the floor and move your right knee toward your chest. Return to the starting position, and repeat with your left leg. Alternate legs, moving quickly.

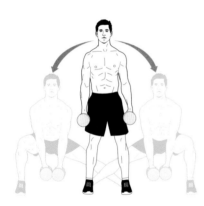

### LOW SIDE-TO-SIDE LUNGE

Stand with your feet shoulder-width apart and clasp your hands in front of your chest (or hold dumbbells, as illustrated). Shift your weight to your right leg and lower your body, bending your right knee and pushing your butt back. Keep your left leg straight and left foot flat on the floor. Without raising yourself all the way to standing, shift the movement to the left. Alternate back and forth. (NOTE: Be sure to push your hips back as you lower down and engage your core to keep your upper body vertical.)

### SINGLE-LEG, SINGLE-ARM PLANK

Assume a pushup position but with your weight on your forearms. Brace your abs, clench your glutes, and keep your body straight from head to heels. Raise your left leg and extend your right arm in front of you. Hold for 5 seconds, then lower your arm and leg and raise your right leg/left arm for 5 seconds. Alternate for the allotted time.

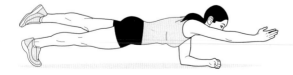

## THIRD 10

**1 MINUTE:** Rest.

**9 MINUTES:** Perform each exercise for 1 minute, cycling through the set three times.

### PRONE COBRA

Lie facedown on the floor with your legs straight and your arms at your sides, palms down. Contract your glutes and lift your head, chest, arms, and legs off the floor. Simultaneously rotate your arms so your thumbs point toward the ceiling. Your hips should be the only part of your body touching the floor. Hold for a 5 count, then return to the starting position. Perform as many reps as you can in the allotted time.

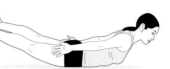

### BURPEE WITH PUSHUP

Stand with your feet shoulder-width apart. Squat as deeply as you can and place your hands on the floor. Kick back into a pushup position. Do 1 pushup. Bring your legs back to a squat and jump up. Land and repeat.

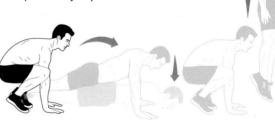

### REVERSE LUNGE AND REACHBACK

Stand tall with your feet hip-width apart. Step backward with your right leg, and lower your body until your left knee is bent at least 90 degrees. Once in this position, reach your arms up and back toward your left shoulder. Press back up to a standing position, and then step back with your left leg, this time reaching toward your right.

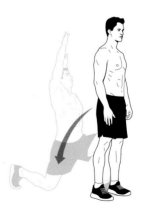

# DO IT WITH DUMBBELLS

A couple of hunks of iron can do your body wonders. I've limited the fitness equipment in this book to just dumbbells (and a bench, box, or step) so you wouldn't need an entire gym to do the workouts but also because I like the beauty of simplicity. These workouts will give you a serious challenge and serious results—all from two simple weights.

# Do It with Dumbbells #1

## FIRST 10

**3 MINUTES:** Do the Dynamic Warmup (page 125).

**1 MINUTE:** Rest.

**6 MINUTES:** Perform each exercise for 1 minute, cycling through the set two times.

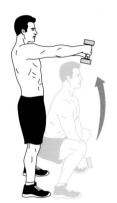

### DUMBBELL SWING

(NOTE: You can also use a kettlebell for this exercise.) Using both hands, hold a dumbbell by one end with your arms hanging straight down in front of you. Stand with your feet hip-width apart, chest up, and shoulders back. Bend your knees slightly and push the weight back between your legs, then explode forward and upward with your hips to propel the weight out in front of you. Brace your core and squeeze your glutes as you swing the weight up, using momentum, until the weight is at chest height. In a smooth motion, swing the weight back down between your legs. Repeat.

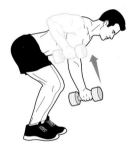

### DUMBBELL ROW

Holding a dumbbell in each hand, bend at your hips and knees and lower your torso until it's nearly parallel to the floor. Let the dumbbells hang at arm's length. Now pull the dumbbells up to the sides of your chest. Pause, then slowly lower them.

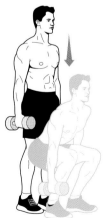

### SUITCASE DEADLIFT

Using a neutral grip, hold a dumbbell in your right hand at arm's length next to your thigh (as if you're holding a suitcase). Stand with your feet hip-width apart and your knees slightly bent. Keeping your chest up, push your hips back and lower your body until the dumbbell is at mid-shin level. Pause, then return to the starting position. Keep the dumbbell close to your side throughout the move. Halfway through the allotted time, switch sides.

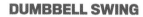

## SECOND 10

**1 MINUTE:** Rest.

**9 MINUTES:** Perform each exercise for 1 minute, cycling through the set three times.

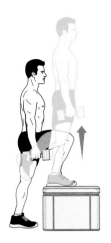

### DUMBBELL STEPUP

Grab a pair of dumbbells and hold them at arm's length at your sides. Stand facing a bench or step and place your right foot on it. Press your right heel into the bench and push your body up until your right leg is straight and you're standing on one leg. (Keep your left foot elevated.) Now lower your body until your left foot touches the floor. That's 1 rep. Repeat for half the allotted time, then switch legs.

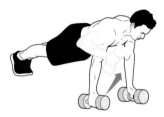

### PUSHUP-POSITION HAMMER CURL

Grip a pair of dumbbells and assume a pushup position with your palms facing each other. Brace your core and glutes. Without moving your upper arm, curl the weight in your right hand toward your right shoulder. Lower it, then repeat with your left arm. Alternate for the allotted time.

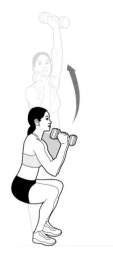

### DUMBBELL SQUAT TO ALTERNATING SHOULDER PRESS AND TWIST

Stand with your feet shoulder-width apart and hold a pair of dumbbells next to your shoulders, elbows bent and palms facing in. Push your hips back and squat until your thighs are parallel to the floor. Push back up, rotating your torso to the right and pivoting on your left foot as you press the dumbbell in your left hand above your shoulder. Lower the weight and rotate back to center. Repeat, alternating sides throughout the allotted time.

## THIRD 10

**1 MINUTE:** Rest.

**9 MINUTES:** Perform each exercise for 1 minute, cycling through the set three times.

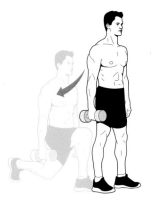

### WAITER'S WALK

Stand straight with a dumbbell in your right hand. Raise the dumbbell over your head (like a waiter carrying a tray). Now walk forward and backward (you can mix it up). Shift the weight to your left hand halfway through the allotted time. If you can walk for longer than 1 minute, use a heavier dumbbell.

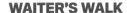

### DUMBBELL OFFSET REVERSE LUNGE

Hold a dumbbell in your right hand next to your side. Step back with your right foot and slowly lower your body until your front knee is bent 90 degrees. Pause, then push back up to the starting position. Halfway through the allotted time, switch sides and legs.

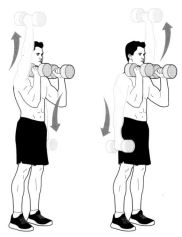

### ALTERNATING DUMBBELL CURL AND PRESS

Stand with a pair of dumbbells just outside your shoulders, arms bent, and palms facing each other. Press the right dumbbell overhead as you lower the left one to your side. Reverse the move as you return to the starting position, then press the left dumbbell overhead and lower the right. Alternate for the allotted time.

# Do It with Dumbbells #2

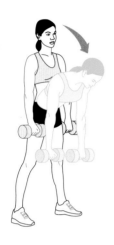

**3 MINUTES:** Do the Dynamic Warmup (page 125).

**1 MINUTE:** Rest.

**6 MINUTES:** Perform each exercise for 1 minute, cycling through the set two times.

## DUMBBELL STRAIGHT-LEG DEADLIFT

Hold a pair of dumbbells in front of your thighs with your feet hip-width apart and your knees slightly bent. Hinge forward at your hips, lowering your torso until it's nearly parallel to the floor. Pause, then return to the starting position.

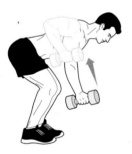

## DUMBBELL ROW

Holding a dumbbell in each hand, bend at your hips and knees and lower your torso until it's nearly parallel to the floor. Let the dumbbells hang at arm's length. Now pull the dumbbells up to the sides of your chest. Pause, then slowly lower them.

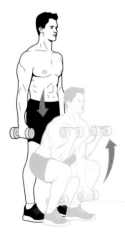

## SQUAT CONCENTRATION CURL

Hold a pair of light dumbbells and stand with your feet about shoulder-width apart and your toes pointed out slightly. Push your hips back and squat until your thighs are parallel to the floor. Keeping your weight on your heels, your elbows pressed against your inner thighs, and your palms facing each other, curl and lower the weights for the allotted time. Do it one arm at a time to add an element of instability and challenge your core.

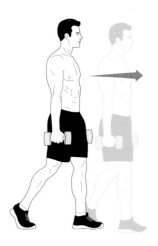

## SECOND 10

**1 MINUTE:** Rest.

**9 MINUTES:** Perform each exercise for 1 minute, cycling through the set three times.

### FARMER'S WALK

Grab a pair of heavy dumbbells and let them hang naturally at arm's length by your sides, holding them as tightly as possible. Now walk for as long as you can before your grip starts to fail. (Walk forward and backward for equal amounts of time; for an added challenge, walk on your toes to target your calves.) If you can walk for longer than 1 minute, try heavier weights.

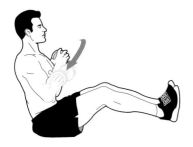

### DUMBBELL RUSSIAN TWIST

Sit on the floor, holding a dumbbell in front of your chest with both hands. Lean your torso back slightly and raise your feet off the floor. Without moving your torso, rotate the weight to your right and then to your left. Move back and forth quickly throughout the allotted time.

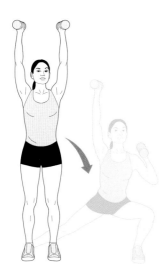

### DUMBBELL SIDE LUNGE AND PRESS

Stand with your feet hip-width apart, pressing a pair of dumbbells over your head so that your arms are straight. Brace your core, then step to the left and lower your body into a side lunge as you lower the left dumbbell to your shoulder. Keep your torso as upright as possible. Reverse the movement and push yourself back to the starting position. Alternate left and right for the allotted time.

## THIRD 10

**1 MINUTE:** Rest.

**9 MINUTES:** Perform each exercise for 1 minute, cycling through the set three times.

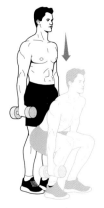

### SUITCASE DEADLIFT

Using a neutral grip, hold a dumbbell in your right hand at arm's length next to your thigh (as if you're holding a suitcase). Stand with your feet hip-width apart and your knees slightly bent. Keeping your chest up, push your hips back and lower your body until the dumbbell is at mid-shin level. Pause, then return to the starting position. Keep the dumbbell close to your side throughout the move. Halfway through the allotted time, switch sides.

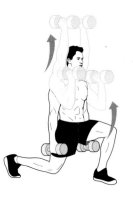

### DUMBBELL LUNGE, CURL, AND PRESS

Stand holding a pair of dumbbells at your sides, palms facing each other and feet hip-width apart. Keeping your torso upright, step forward with your left foot and lower your body until your left knee is bent 90 degrees. Hold that position and curl the dumbbells to your shoulders. Then press the dumbbells above your shoulders until your arms are straight. Lower the dumbbells back to your sides, and then push yourself back to the starting position. Alternate legs for the allotted time.

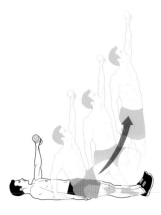

### TURKISH GET-UP

Lie on your back with your right arm by your side and a dumbbell or kettlebell in your left hand above your chest. Now roll onto your right side, prop up on your right forearm, and push yourself into a half kneel by threading your right leg behind your left. Stand up to complete the move. Reverse it to return to the starting position. Switch sides halfway through your time.

# Do It with Dumbbells #3

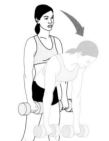

**3 MINUTES:** Do the Dynamic Warmup (page 125).

**1 MINUTE:** Rest.

**6 MINUTES:** Perform each exercise for 1 minute, cycling through the set two times.

### DUMBBELL STRAIGHT-LEG DEADLIFT

Hold a pair of dumbbells in front of your thighs with your feet hip-width apart and your knees slightly bent. Hinge forward at your hips, lowering your torso until it's nearly parallel to the floor. Pause, then return to the starting position.

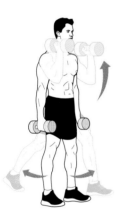

### SPLIT-JACK CURL

Hold a pair of dumbbells at your sides, palms in, feet hip-width apart. Jump into a split stance—left leg forward—while curling the weights to your shoulders. Return to the starting position and repeat, landing with your right leg forward. Alternate for the allotted time.

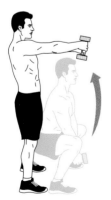

### DUMBBELL SWING

(NOTE: You can also use a kettlebell for this exercise.) Using both hands, hold a dumbbell by one end with your arms hanging straight down in front of you. Stand with your feet hip-width apart, chest up, and shoulders back. Bend your knees slightly and push the weight back between your legs, then explode forward and upward with your hips to propel the weight out in front of you. Brace your core and squeeze your glutes as you swing the weight up, using momentum, until the weight is at chest height. In a smooth motion, swing the weight back down between your legs. Repeat.

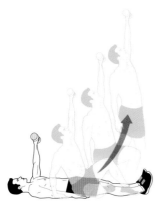

## SECOND 10

**1 MINUTE:** Rest.

**9 MINUTES:** Perform each exercise for 1 minute, cycling through the set three times.

### TURKISH GET-UP

Lie on your back with your right arm by your side and a dumbbell or kettlebell in your left hand above your chest. Now roll onto your right side, prop up on your right forearm, and push yourself into a half kneel by threading your right leg behind your left. Stand up to complete the move. Reverse it to return to the starting position. Switch sides halfway through your time.

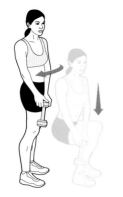

### DUMBBELL ROTATIONAL DEADLIFT

Stand tall and use both hands to grasp a dumbbell by its end, letting it hang at arm's length in front of your waist. Now rotate your hips to the right so the weight is hanging next to your right thigh. Next, keep your back naturally arched as you bend your knees and hips and lower the weight to the front of your right shin. Push your hips forward, raise your torso, and stand; then rotate your torso all the way to the left to repeat the move on that side.

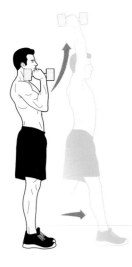

### WAITER'S WALK

Stand straight with a dumbbell in your right hand. Raise the dumbbell over your head (like a waiter carrying a tray). Now walk forward and backward (you can mix it up). Shift the weight to your left hand halfway through the allotted time. If you can walk for longer than 1 minute, use a heavier dumbbell.

## THIRD 10

**1 MINUTE:** Rest.

**9 MINUTES:** Perform each exercise for 1 minute, cycling through the set three times.

### DUMBBELL HAMMER CURL AND PRESS

Standing with your feet shoulder-width apart, hold a pair of dumbbells at arm's length by your sides, palms facing each other. Without moving your upper arms, curl the weights to your shoulders, then press them overhead until your arms are straight. Reverse the move to return to the starting position.

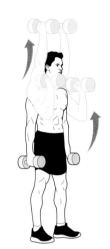

### "DEATH CRAWL" WITH DUMBBELL JUMP SQUAT

Assume a pushup position, grasping one dumbbell in each hand. Do a pushup, then row the dumbbell in your right hand up to the side of your chest and lower it to the floor. Do the same with your left arm. Now "walk" the dumbbell in your left hand forward one step, followed by the one in your right. Next bring your left foot, then right foot, forward. Move ahead three steps with each hand. Keep your core tense and back straight throughout the movement. Then stand up and do 3 dumbbell jump squats (holding the dumbbells at your sides, bend your knees and squat, then jump up explosively). That's 1 rep. Alternate walking forward and backward. Do as much as you can in the allotted time.

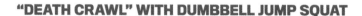

### DUMBBELL COMPASS LUNGE AND SHOULDER PRESS

Stand, holding a pair of dumbbells at your shoulders. Step forward (or "north") with your right leg and lower your body until the top of your right thigh is parallel to the floor and your left knee comes close to the floor. At the same time, press the dumbbells overhead. Push back to standing as you lower the dumbbells to your shoulders. Repeat the exercise while hitting points on the compass (northeast, east, etc.). (NOTE: Northern lunges are forward, southern are reverse.) When you hit "due south," switch legs and continue until you reach north again. Do as much as you can in the allotted time.

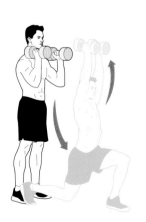

# Do It with Dumbbells #4

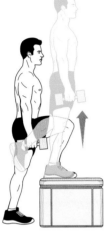

## FIRST 10

**3 MINUTES:** Do the Dynamic Warmup (page 125).

**1 MINUTE:** Rest.

**6 MINUTES:** Perform each exercise for 1 minute, cycling through the set two times.

### DUMBBELL STEPUP

Grab a pair of dumbbells and hold them at arm's length at your sides. Stand facing a bench or step and place your right foot on it. Press your right heel into the bench and push your body up until your right leg is straight and you're standing on one leg. (Keep your left foot elevated.) Now lower your body until your left foot touches the floor. That's 1 rep. Repeat for half the allotted time, then switch legs.

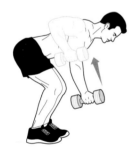

### DUMBBELL ROW

Holding a dumbbell in each hand, bend at your hips and knees and lower your torso until it's nearly parallel to the floor. Let the dumbbells hang at arm's length. Now pull the dumbbells up to the sides of your chest. Pause, then slowly lower them.

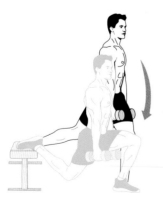

### DUMBBELL BULGARIAN SPLIT SQUAT

Hold a pair of dumbbells at arm's length next to your hips. Stand in a staggered stance and place the top of your back foot on a bench, step, or chair. Keeping your torso upright, bend your front knee and lower your body as far as you can. Pause, then push back to the starting position. Halfway through the allotted time, switch legs.

## SECOND 10

**1 MINUTE:** Rest.

**9 MINUTES:** Perform each exercise for 1 minute, cycling through the set three times.

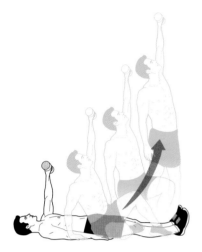

### TURKISH GET-UP

Lie on your back with your right arm by your side and a dumbbell or kettlebell in your left hand above your chest. Now roll onto your right side, prop up on your right forearm, and push yourself into a half kneel by threading your right leg behind your left. Stand up to complete the move. Reverse it to return to the starting position. Switch sides halfway through your time.

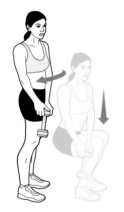

### DUMBBELL ROTATIONAL DEADLIFT

Stand tall and use both hands to grasp a dumbbell by its end, letting it hang at arm's length in front of your waist. Now rotate your hips to the right so your right foot is forward and the weight is hanging next to your right thigh. Next, keep your back naturally arched as you bend your knees and hips and lower the weight to the front of your right shin. Push your hips forward, raise your torso, and stand; then rotate your torso all the way to the left to repeat the move on that side.

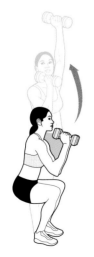

### DUMBBELL SQUAT TO ALTERNATING SHOULDER PRESS AND TWIST

Stand with your feet shoulder-width apart and hold a pair of dumbbells next to your shoulders, elbows bent and palms facing in. Push your hips back and squat until your thighs are parallel to the floor. Push back up, rotating your torso to the right and pivoting on your left foot as you press the dumbbell in your left hand above your shoulder. Lower the weight and rotate back to center. Repeat, alternating sides throughout the allotted time.

## THIRD 10

**1 MINUTE:** Rest.

**9 MINUTES:** Perform each exercise for 1 minute, cycling through the set three times.

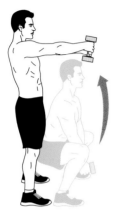

### DUMBBELL SWING

(NOTE: You can also use a kettlebell for this exercise.) Using both hands, hold a dumbbell by one end with your arms hanging straight down in front of you. Stand with your feet hip-width apart, chest up, and shoulders back. Bend your knees slightly and push the weight back between your legs, then explode forward and upward with your hips to propel the weight out in front of you. Brace your core and squeeze your glutes as you swing the weight up, using momentum, until the weight is at chest height. In a smooth motion, swing the weight back down between your legs and repeat.

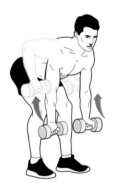

### DUMBBELL STRAIGHT-LEG DEADLIFT AND ROW

Stand with your knees slightly bent and hold a pair of dumbbells at arm's length in front of your thighs. Without rounding your lower back or changing the bend in your knees, bend at your hips and lower your torso until it's nearly parallel to the floor. Without moving your torso, pull the dumbbells up to the sides of your chest. Pause, then lower the dumbbells. Raise your torso back to the starting position.

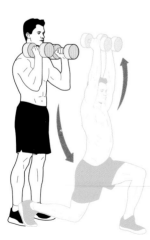

### DUMBBELL COMPASS LUNGE AND SHOULDER PRESS

Stand, holding a pair of dumbbells at your shoulders. Step forward (or "north") with your right leg and lower your body until the top of your right thigh is parallel to the floor and your left knee comes close to the floor. At the same time, press the dumbbells overhead. Push back to standing as you lower the dumbbells to your shoulders. Repeat the exercise while hitting points on the compass (northeast, east, etc.). (NOTE: Northern lunges are forward, southern are reverse.) When you hit "due south," switch legs and continue until you reach north again. Do as much as you can in the allotted time.

# Do It with Dumbbells #5

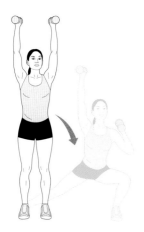

## FIRST 10

**3 MINUTES:** Do the Dynamic Warmup (page 125).

**1 MINUTE:** Rest.

**6 MINUTES:** Perform each exercise for 1 minute, cycling through the set two times.

### DUMBBELL SIDE LUNGE AND PRESS

Stand with your feet hip-width apart, pressing a pair of dumbbells over your head so that your arms are straight. Brace your core, then step to the left and lower your body into a side lunge as you lower the left dumbbell to your shoulder. Keep your torso as upright as possible. Reverse the movement and push yourself back to the starting position. Alternate left and right for the allotted time.

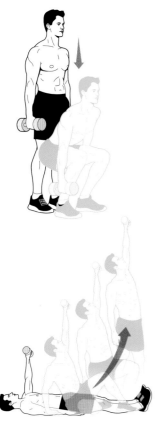

### SUITCASE DEADLIFT

Using a neutral grip, hold a dumbbell in your right hand at arm's length next to your thigh (as if you're holding a suitcase). Stand with your feet hip-width apart and your knees slightly bent. Keeping your chest up, push your hips back and lower your body until the dumbbell is at mid-shin level. Pause, then return to the starting position. Keep the dumbbell close to your side throughout the move. Halfway through the allotted time, switch sides.

### TURKISH GET-UP

Lie on on your back with your right arm by your side and a dumbbell or kettlebell in your left hand above your chest. Now roll onto your right side, prop up on your right forearm, and push yourself into a half kneel by threading your right leg behind your left. Stand up to complete the move. Reverse it to return to the starting position. Switch sides halfway through your time.

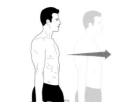
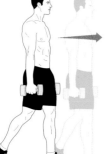

## SECOND 10

**1 MINUTE:** Rest.

**9 MINUTES:** Perform each exercise for 1 minute, cycling through the set three times.

### FARMER'S WALK

Grab a pair of heavy dumbbells and let them hang naturally at arm's length by your sides, holding them as tightly as possible. Now walk for as long as you can before your grip starts to fail. (Walk forward and backward for equal amounts of time; for an added challenge, walk on your toes to target your calves.) If you can walk for longer than 1 minute, try heavier weights.

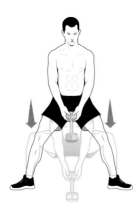

### DUMBBELL SUMO SQUAT AND HOLD

Hold a dumbbell by its end in front of your waist and stand with your feet twice shoulder-width apart. Now lower your body until your thighs are parallel to the floor. Hold the position for as long as you can, up to 30 seconds, and then return to the starting position. Perform the exercise as many times as you can during the allotted time, based on how long you can hold the down position without breaking form.

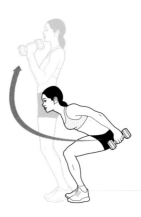

### DUMBBELL SKIER SWING

Holding a pair of dumbbells at arm's length next to your sides, stand with your knees slightly bent. Without rounding your lower back, bend at your hips as you simultaneously swing your arms backward. Now explosively thrust your hips forward and raise your torso until you're standing upright, while allowing your momentum to swing the weights up to chest level. (Don't actively lift the weights.) Swing back and forth for the allotted time.

## THIRD 10

**1 MINUTE:** Rest.

**9 MINUTES:** Perform each exercise for 1 minute, cycling through the set three times.

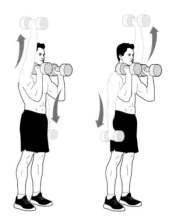

## ALTERNATING DUMBBELL CURL AND PRESS

Stand with a pair of dumbbells just outside your shoulders, arms bent, and palms facing each other. Press the right dumbbell overhead as you lower the left one to your side. Reverse the move as you return to the starting position, then press the left dumbbell overhead and lower the right. Alternate for the allotted time.

## DUMBBELL STEPUP

Grab a pair of dumbbells and hold them at arm's length at your sides. Stand facing a bench or step and place your right foot on it. Press your right heel into the bench and push your body up until your right leg is straight and you're standing on one leg. (Keep your left foot elevated.) Now lower your body until your left foot touches the floor. That's 1 rep. Repeat for half the allotted time, then switch legs.

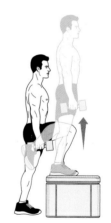

## "DEATH CRAWL" WITH DUMBBELL JUMP SQUAT

Assume a pushup position, grasping one dumbbell in each hand. Do a pushup, then row the dumbbell in your right hand up to the side of your chest and lower it to the floor. Do the same with your left arm. Now "walk" the dumbbell in your left hand forward one step, followed by the one in your right. Next bring your left foot, then right foot, forward. Move ahead three steps with each hand. Keep your core tense and back straight throughout the movement. Then stand up and do 3 dumbbell jump squats (holding the dumbbells at your sides, bend your knees and squat, then jump up explosively). That's 1 rep. Alternate walking forward and backward. Do as much as you can in the allotted time.

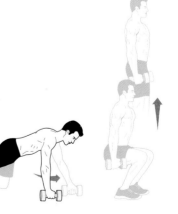

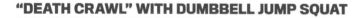

# LOWER-BODY WORKOUTS

Some of your body's biggest muscles reside in your lower body. Some, like the iliopsoas, help your lower body get along with your upper body. And glutes? Well, I've always said that a strong butt is the key to a happy life. These workouts will build an amazingly powerful lower body. And that will help every movement you make—adding power, flexibility, and a serious spring to your step.

# Lower Body #1

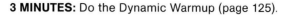

**FIRST 10**

**3 MINUTES:** Do the Dynamic Warmup (page 125).

**1 MINUTE:** Rest.

**6 MINUTES:** Perform each exercise for 1 minute, cycling through the set two times.

### DUMBBELL STEPUP

Grab a pair of dumbbells and hold them at arm's length at your sides. Stand facing a bench or step and place your right foot on it. Press your right heel into the bench and push your body up until your right leg is straight and you're standing on one leg. (Keep your left foot elevated.) Now lower your body until your left foot touches the floor. That's 1 rep. Repeat for half the allotted time, then switch legs.

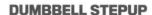

### DUMBBELL SUMO SQUAT AND HOLD

Hold a dumbbell by its end in front of your waist and stand with your feet twice shoulder-width apart. Now lower your body until your thighs are parallel to the floor. Hold the position for as long as you can, up to 30 seconds, and then return to the starting position. Perform the exercise as many times as you can during the allotted time, based on how long you can hold the down position without breaking form.

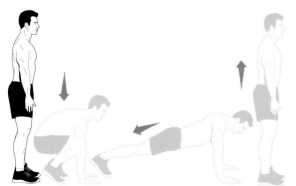

### BURPEE

Stand with your feet shoulder-width apart. Squat as deeply as you can and place your hands on the floor. Kick into a pushup position. Bring your legs back to a squat and jump up, land, and repeat.

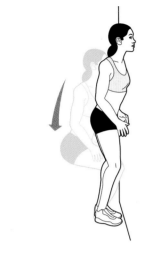

## SECOND 10

**1 MINUTE:** Rest.

**9 MINUTES:** Perform each exercise for 1 minute, cycling through the set three times.

### RUSSIAN WALL SQUAT

Face a wall with your feet shoulder-width apart and toes touching the wall. Keep your arms by your sides and squat until your thighs are parallel to the floor. Pause, then return to the starting position.

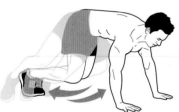

### MOGUL JUMP

Get on all fours and lift your knees a few inches off the floor so your weight is on your hands and the balls of your feet. Keeping your arms straight and legs together, hop, rotating your knees and feet to the right. Now hop as you rotate your knees and feet to the left. That's 1 rep. Alternate sides for the allotted time.

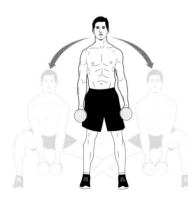

### LOW SIDE-TO-SIDE LUNGE

Stand with your feet shoulder-width apart and clasp your hands in front of your chest (or hold dumbbells, as illustrated). Shift your weight to your right leg and lower your body, bending your right knee and pushing your butt back. Keep your left leg straight and left foot flat on the floor. Without raising yourself all the way to standing, shift the movement to the left. Alternate back and forth. (NOTE: Be sure to push your hips back as you lower down and engage your core to keep your upper body vertical.)

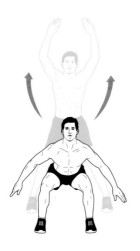

## THIRD 10

**1 MINUTE:** Rest.

**9 MINUTES:** Perform each exercise for 1 minute, cycling through the set three times.

### STAR JUMP

With your feet about shoulder-width apart, squat so your hands move down to the floor near your feet. Then, in one movement, jump up into the air and spread your arms and legs out as wide as you possibly can. Return to the starting position and repeat.

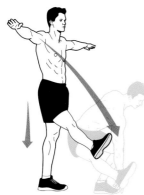

### SINGLE-LEG TOE TOUCHES

Stand on your left leg with your right leg out in front of you, raised off the floor. Extend your arms straight out at your sides at shoulder height. Bend your left leg at the knee and squat down to touch your right hand to the toe of your left foot, then come back up. Repeat with your right leg and continue, alternating for the allotted time.

### HIGH KNEES

(NOTE: If you have room, such as if you are working outdoors, substitute regular running sprints.) Sprint in place, bringing your knees up to your chest. Keep your back straight as you pump your arms and drive your hands past your hips in time with your legs for the allotted time.

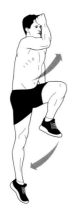

# Lower Body #2

**3 MINUTES:** Do the Dynamic Warmup (page 125).

**1 MINUTE:** Rest.

**6 MINUTES:** Perform each exercise for 1 minute, cycling through the set two times.

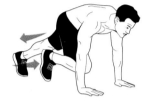

## MOUNTAIN CLIMBER

Assume a pushup position. Your body should form a straight line from your head to your ankles. Without allowing your lower-back posture to change, lift your right foot off the floor and move your right knee toward your chest. Return to the starting position, and repeat with your left leg. Alternate legs, moving quickly.

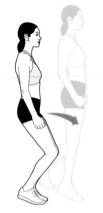

## MULTIDIRECTIONAL HOP

Stand with your knees slightly bent. Jump forward 12 inches and land on your right foot. Hop backward to the starting position, landing on both feet. Repeat on your left foot. Next do the sequence going sideways. Continue throughout the allotted time. (Hold a dumbbell in front of your chest with both hands for an added challenge.)

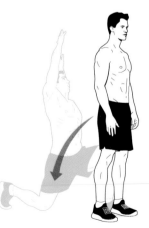

## REVERSE LUNGE AND REACHBACK

Stand tall with your feet hip-width apart. Step backward with your right leg, and lower your body until your left knee is bent at least 90 degrees. Once in this position, reach your arms up and back toward your left shoulder. Press back up to a standing position, and then step back with your left leg, this time reaching toward your right.

## SECOND 10

**1 MINUTE:** Rest.

**9 MINUTES:** Perform each exercise for 1 minute, cycling through the set three times.

### SKATER HOP

This exercise mimics the explosive side-to-side movements of speed skaters. Stand on your right foot with your right knee slightly bent, and place your left foot back behind your right ankle. Bend your right knee and lower your body into a partial squat. Then explosively bound to the left by jumping off your right foot. Land on your left foot and bring your right foot back behind your left foot. Reach your right hand toward your left foot. Hop back to the right, landing on your right foot and reaching for the floor with your left hand (touch the floor if you're able). Repeat, alternating sides.

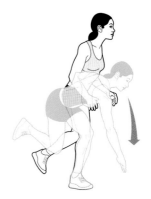

### SUMO BURPEE

Stand with your feet several inches wider than your shoulders, then squat (like a sumo wrestler) and place your hands on the floor in front of you. Kick your legs back into a pushup position, quickly bring your legs back to a squat, and jump up, throwing your hands above your head. Land and repeat.

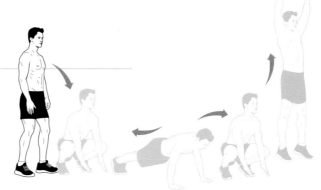

### DUMBBELL STEPUP

Grab a pair of dumbbells and hold them at arm's length at your sides. Stand facing a bench or step and place your right foot on it. Press your right heel into the bench and push your body up until your right leg is straight and you're standing on one leg. (Keep your left foot elevated.) Now lower your body until your left foot touches the floor. That's 1 rep. Repeat for half the allotted time, then switch legs.

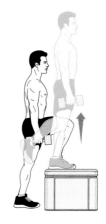

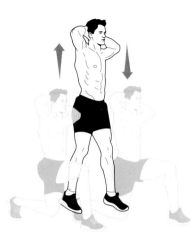

## THIRD 10

**1 MINUTE:** Rest.

**9 MINUTES:** Perform each exercise for 1 minute, cycling through the set three times.

### BODYWEIGHT SPLIT JUMP

Place your hands behind your head and assume a staggered stance, right leg forward. Slowly lower your body as far as you can, then jump with enough force to propel both feet off the floor. Land with your left leg forward. That's 1 rep. Alternate back and forth for the allotted time.

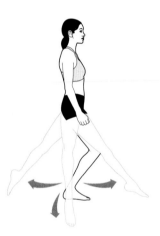

### THREE-POINT BALANCE TOUCH

Standing on your left leg with your knee slightly bent and chest up, perform a quarter squat. Your right leg (the nonbalancing leg) will perform the following three actions while the rest of the body remains still.

A. Reach your right foot as far forward as possible and gently tap the floor, then return to the starting position.

B. Next reach your right foot out to the right as far as possible, tap the floor with your toes, and return to the starting position.

C. Finally, reach your right foot as far back behind you as possible, touch the floor with your toes, and return to the starting position.

That's 1 repetition. Alternate legs for the allotted time. The deeper you squat, the harder this exercise becomes.

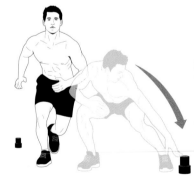

### SHUTTLE RUN

Place two cones or other kinds of markers 10 to 25 yards apart (depending on how much room you have). Sprint from one to the other and back.

# Lower Body #3

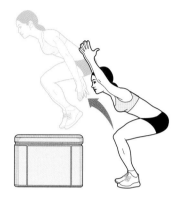

## FIRST 10

**3 MINUTES:** Do the Dynamic Warmup (page 125).

**1 MINUTE:** Rest.

**6 MINUTES:** Perform each exercise for 1 minute, cycling through the set two times.

### BOX JUMP

Stand in front of a knee-high box, bench, or step with your arms raised. Drive your arms down, dip your knees, and jump onto the box. Step down.

### THREE-POINT BALANCE TOUCH

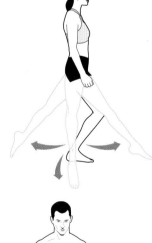

Standing on your left leg with your knee slightly bent and chest up, perform a quarter squat. Your right leg (the nonbalancing leg) will perform the following three actions while the rest of your body remains still.

A. Reach your right foot as far forward as possible and gently tap the floor, then return to the starting position.

B. Next reach your right foot out to the right as far as possible, tap the floor with your toes, and return to the starting position.

C. Finally, reach your right foot as far back behind you as possible, touch the floor with your toes, and return to the starting position.

That's 1 repetition. Alternate legs for the allotted time. The deeper you squat, the harder this exercise becomes.

### DUMBBELL SUMO SQUAT AND HOLD

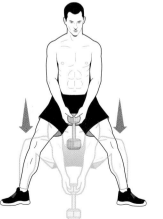

Hold a dumbbell by its end in front of your waist and stand with your feet twice shoulder-width apart. Now lower your body until your thighs are parallel to the floor. Hold the position for as long as you can, up to 30 seconds, and then return to the starting position. Perform the exercise as many times as you can during the allotted time, based on how long you can hold the down position without breaking form.

## SECOND 10

**1 MINUTE:** Rest.

**9 MINUTES:** Perform each exercise for 1 minute, cycling through the set three times.

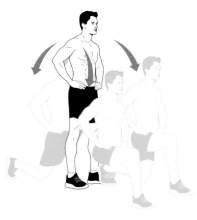

### COMPASS LUNGE

Stand with your feet hip-width apart. Step forward (or "north") with your right leg and lower your body until the top of your right thigh is parallel to the floor and your left knee comes close to the floor. Push back to standing and repeat the exercise while hitting points on the compass (northeast, east, etc.). (NOTE: Northern lunges are forward; southern are reverse; east and west are side lunges.) When you hit "due south," switch legs and continue until you reach north again. Do as much as you can in the allotted time.

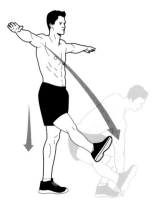

### SINGLE-LEG TOE TOUCHES

Stand on your left leg with your right leg out in front of you, raised off the floor. Extend your arms straight out at your sides at shoulder height. Bend your left leg at the knee and squat down to touch your right hand to the toe of your left foot, then come back up. Repeat with your right leg and continue, alternating for the allotted time.

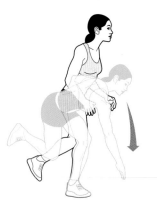

### SKATER HOP

This exercise mimics the explosive side-to-side movements of speed skaters. Stand on your right foot with your right knee slightly bent, and place your left foot back behind your right ankle. Bend your right knee and lower your body into a partial squat. Then explosively bound to the left by jumping off your right foot. Land on your left foot and bring your right foot back behind your left foot. Reach your right hand toward your left foot. Hop back to the right, landing on your right foot and reaching for the floor with your left hand (touch the floor if you're able). Repeat, alternating sides.

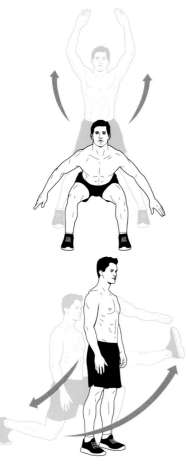

## THIRD 10

**1 MINUTE:** Rest.

**9 MINUTES:** Perform each exercise for 1 minute, cycling through the set three times.

### STAR JUMP

With your feet about shoulder-width apart, squat so your hands move down to the floor near your feet. Then, in one movement, jump up into the air and spread your arms and legs out as wide as you possibly can. Return to the starting position and repeat.

### REVERSE LUNGE WITH TOE TOUCH

Stand with your feet hip-width apart. Step back with your right leg and lower your body until your knee almost touches the floor. Stand up, swing your right leg as high as you can, and touch your toes with your left hand. Alternate sides for the allotted time.

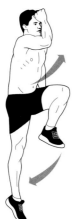

### HIGH KNEES

(NOTE: If you have room, such as if you are working outdoors, substitute regular running sprints.) Sprint in place, bringing your knees up to your chest. Keep your back straight as you pump your arms and drive your hands past your hips in time with your legs for the allotted time.

# Lower Body #4

**3 MINUTES:** Do the Dynamic Warmup (page 125).

**1 MINUTE:** Rest.

**6 MINUTES:** Perform each exercise for 1 minute, cycling through the set two times.

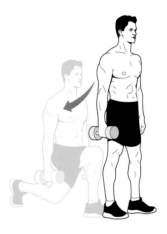

### DUMBBELL OFFSET REVERSE LUNGE

Hold a dumbbell in your right hand next to your side. Step back with your right foot and slowly lower your body until your front knee is bent 90 degrees. Pause, then push back up to the starting position. Halfway through the allotted time, switch sides and legs.

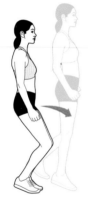

### MULTIDIRECTIONAL HOP

Stand with your knees slightly bent. Jump forward 12 inches and land on your right foot. Hop backward to the starting position, landing on both feet. Repeat on your left foot. Next do the sequence going sideways. Continue throughout the allotted time. (Hold a dumbbell in front of your chest with both hands for an added challenge.)

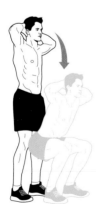

### BODYWEIGHT SQUAT

Stand with your hands on the back of your head and your feet shoulder-width apart. Lower your body until your thighs are parallel to the floor. Pause, then return to the starting position. Repeat for the allotted time.

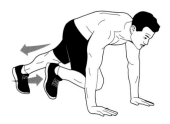

## SECOND 10

**1 MINUTE:** Rest.

**9 MINUTES:** Perform each exercise for 1 minute, cycling through the set three times.

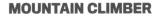

### MOUNTAIN CLIMBER

Assume a pushup position. Your body should form a straight line from your head to your ankles. Without allowing your lower-back posture to change, lift your right foot off the floor and move your right knee toward your chest. Return to the starting position, and repeat with your left leg. Alternate legs, moving quickly.

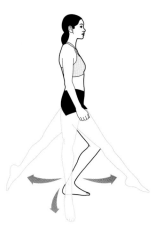

### THREE-POINT BALANCE TOUCH

Standing on your left leg with your knee slightly bent and chest up, perform a quarter squat. Your right leg (the nonbalancing leg) will perform the following three actions while the rest of your body remains still.

A. Reach your right foot as far forward as possible and gently tap the floor, then return to the starting position.

B. Next reach your right foot out to the right as far as possible, tap the floor with your toes, and return to the starting position.

C. Finally, reach your right foot as far back behind you as possible, touch the floor with your toes, and return to the starting position.

That's 1 repetition. Alternate legs for the allotted time. The deeper you squat, the harder this exercise becomes.

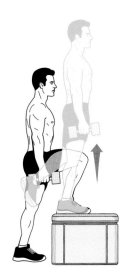

### DUMBBELL STEPUP

Grab a pair of dumbbells and hold them at arm's length at your sides. Stand facing a bench or step and place your right foot on it. Press your right heel into the bench and push your body up until your right leg is straight and you're standing on one leg. (Keep your left foot elevated.) Now lower your body until your left foot touches the floor. That's 1 rep. Repeat for half the allotted time, then switch legs.

## THIRD 10

**1 MINUTE:** Rest.

**9 MINUTES:** Perform each exercise for 1 minute, cycling through the set three times.

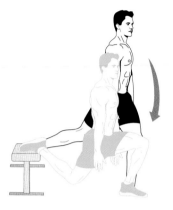

### DUMBBELL BULGARIAN SPLIT SQUAT

Hold a pair of dumbbells at arm's length next to your hips. Stand in a staggered stance and place the top of your back foot on a bench, step, or chair. Keeping your torso upright, bend your front knee and lower your body as far as you can. Pause, then push back to the starting position. Halfway through the allotted time, switch legs.

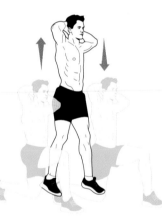

### BODYWEIGHT SPLIT JUMP

Place your hands behind your head and assume a staggered stance, right leg forward. Slowly lower your body as far as you can, then jump with enough force to propel both feet off the floor. Land with your left leg forward. That's 1 rep. Alternate back and forth for the allotted time.

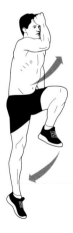

### HIGH KNEES

(NOTE: If you have room, such as if you are working outdoors, substitute regular running sprints.) Sprint in place, bringing your knees up to your chest. Keep your back straight as you pump your arms and drive your hands past your hips in time with your legs for the allotted time.

# Lower Body #5

**3 MINUTES:** Do the Dynamic Warmup (page 125).

**1 MINUTE:** Rest.

**6 MINUTES:** Perform each exercise for 1 minute, cycling through the set two times.

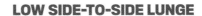
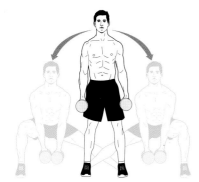

## LOW SIDE-TO-SIDE LUNGE

Stand with your feet shoulder-width apart and clasp your hands in front of your chest (or hold dumbbells, as illustrated). Shift your weight to your right leg and lower your body, bending your right knee and pushing your butt back. Keep your left leg straight and left foot flat on the floor. Without raising yourself all the way to standing, shift the movement to the left. Alternate back and forth. (NOTE: Be sure to push your hips back as you lower down and engage your core to keep your upper body vertical.)

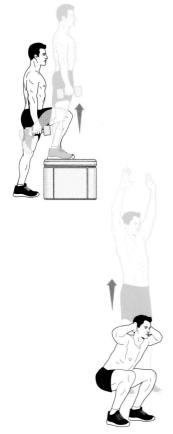

## DUMBBELL STEPUP

Grab a pair of dumbbells and hold them at arm's length at your sides. Stand facing a bench or step and place your right foot on it. Press your right heel into the bench and push your body up until your right leg is straight and you're standing on one leg. (Keep your left foot elevated.) Now lower your body until your left foot touches the floor. That's 1 rep. Repeat for half the allotted time, then switch legs.

## SQUAT JUMP

Start with your feet shoulder-width apart and hands on hips. Now squat with your heels flat and touch the floor with your palms. Jump forcefully, thrusting your arms overhead with palms inward to boost your momentum. Land and immediately begin the next jump.

## SECOND 10

**1 MINUTE:** Rest.

**9 MINUTES:** Perform each exercise for 1 minute, cycling through the set three times.

### BURPEE

Stand with your feet shoulder-width apart. Squat as deeply as you can and place your hands on the floor. Kick into a pushup position. Bring your legs back to a squat and jump up, land, and repeat.

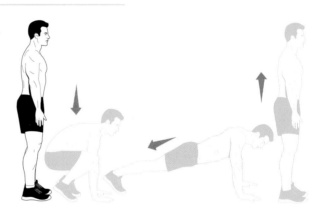

### SINGLE-LEG TOE TOUCHES

Stand on your left leg with your right leg out in front of you, raised off the floor. Extend your arms straight out at your sides at shoulder height. Bend your left leg at the knee and squat down to touch your right hand to the toe of your left foot, then come back up. Repeat with your right leg and continue, alternating for the allotted time.

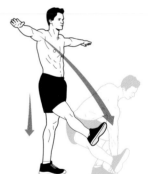

### MULTIDIRECTIONAL HOP

Stand with your knees slightly bent. Jump forward 12 inches and land on your right foot. Hop backward to the starting position, landing on both feet. Repeat on your left foot. Next do the sequence going sideways. Continue throughout the allotted time. (Hold a dumbbell in front of your chest with both hands for an added challenge.)

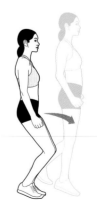

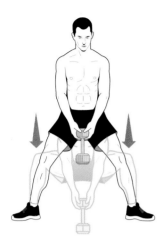

## THIRD 10

**1 MINUTE:** Rest.

**9 MINUTES:** Perform each exercise for 1 minute, cycling through the set three times.

### DUMBBELL SUMO SQUAT AND HOLD

Hold a dumbbell by its end in front of your waist and stand with your feet twice shoulder-width apart. Now lower your body until your thighs are parallel to the floor. Hold the position for as long as you can, up to 30 seconds, and then return to the starting position. Perform the exercise as many times as you can during the allotted time, based on how long you can hold the down position without breaking form.

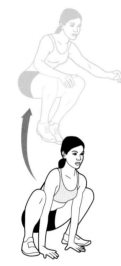

### FROG JUMP

Squat and touch the floor with both hands, keeping your arms straight. Then explode into the air, raising your knees as high as they'll go. Land and immediately begin the next jump.

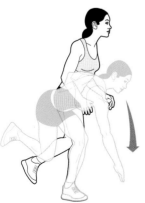

### SKATER HOP

This exercise mimics the explosive side-to-side movements of speed skaters. Stand on your right foot with your right knee slightly bent, and place your left foot back behind your right ankle. Bend your right knee and lower your body into a partial squat. Then explosively bound to the left by jumping off your right foot. Land on your left foot and bring your right foot back behind your left foot. Reach your right hand toward your left foot. Hop back to the right, landing on your right foot and reaching for the floor with your left hand (touch the floor if you're able). Repeat, alternating sides.

# UPPER-BODY WORKOUTS

It's easy to get caught up in the vanity muscles when you talk about the upper body. Show me a man or woman with toned arms and I'll show you a sleeve shortage. Hey, being proud is fine. But these workouts won't just give you those "flex-able" arms. They'll build an upper musculature—arms, shoulders, chest, upper back—that will make you more athletic, give you a more powerful grip, and improve subtler things like posture.

# Upper Body #1

**3 MINUTES:** Do the Dynamic Warmup (page 125).

**1 MINUTE:** Rest.

**6 MINUTES:** Perform each exercise for 1 minute, cycling through the set two times.

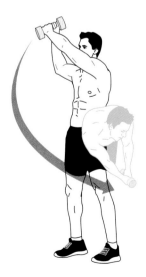

## PUSHUP

Get down on all fours, placing your hands slightly wider than your shoulders. Straighten your arms and legs. Lower your body until your chest nearly touches the floor. Pause, then push yourself back up. Repeat for the allotted time.

## REAR LATERAL RAISE

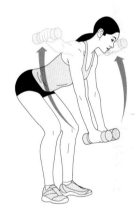

Grab a pair of dumbbells and bend forward at your hips until your torso is nearly parallel to the floor. Set your feet shoulder-width apart. Let the dumbbells hang straight down from your shoulders, your palms facing each other. Without moving your torso, raise your arms straight out to your sides until they're in line with your body. Pause, then slowly return to the starting position.

## DUMBBELL CHOP

Hold a dumbbell with both hands above your right shoulder. Stand with your feet shoulder-width apart. Brace your core and rotate your torso to the right. While keeping your arms straight, swing the dumbbell down and to the outside of your left knee by rotating to the left and bending at your hips. Reverse the movement to return to the starting position. Halfway through the prescribed time, switch sides.

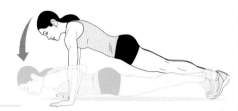

**1 MINUTE:** Rest.

**9 MINUTES:** Perform each exercise for 1 minute, cycling through the set three times.

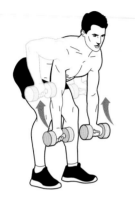

## DUMBBELL STRAIGHT-LEG DEADLIFT AND ROW

Stand with your knees slightly bent and hold a pair of dumbbells at arm's length in front of your thighs. Without rounding your lower back or changing the bend in your knees, bend at your hips and lower your torso until it's nearly parallel to the floor. Without moving your torso, pull the dumbbells up to the sides of your chest. Pause, then lower the dumbbells. Raise your torso back to the starting position.

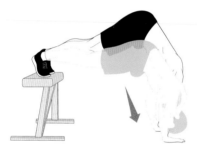

## INVERTED SHOULDER PRESS

Assume a pushup position with your feet on a bench or chair. Push your hips up so your torso is nearly perpendicular to the floor. Your hands should be slightly wider than your shoulders and your arms straight. Without changing your body posture, lower yourself until your head nearly touches the floor. Pause, then return to the starting position.

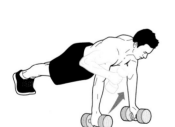

## PUSHUP-POSITION HAMMER CURL

Grip a pair of dumbbells and assume a pushup position with your palms facing each other. Brace your core and glutes. Without moving your upper arm, curl the weight in your right hand toward your right shoulder. Lower it, then repeat with your left arm. Alternate for the allotted time.

**THIRD 10**

**1 MINUTE:** Rest.

**9 MINUTES:** Perform each exercise for 1 minute, cycling through the set three times.

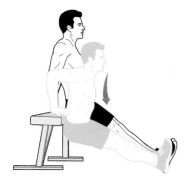

### BENCH DIP

Sit on a flat bench with your hands at your sides on the bench (or grip the sides of a chair seat). Keep your palms on the bench at all times, with your fingers facing forward and your palms down. Walk your feet out a couple of steps until your legs are extended, and lower your body just in front of the bench until your elbows are at 90 degrees. Then press through your palms to raise your body.

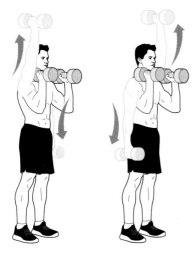

### ALTERNATING DUMBBELL CURL AND PRESS

Stand with a pair of dumbbells just outside your shoulders, arms bent, and palms facing each other. Press the right dumbbell overhead as you lower the left one to your side. Reverse the move as you return to the starting position, then press the left dumbbell overhead and lower the right. Alternate for the allotted time.

### DIVE-BOMBER PUSHUP (SOMETIMES CALLED JUDO PUSHUP)

Begin in the standard pushup position, but move your feet forward and raise your hips so your body almost forms an upside-down V. Keeping your hips elevated, lower your body until your chin nearly touches the floor. Lower your hips until they almost touch the floor, as you simultaneously raise your head and shoulders toward the ceiling. Reverse the movement back to the starting position and repeat.

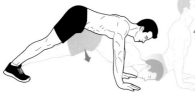

# Upper Body #2

**3 MINUTES:** Do the Dynamic Warmup (page 125).

**1 MINUTE:** Rest.

**6 MINUTES:** Perform each exercise for 1 minute, cycling through the set two times.

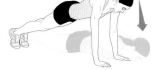

## WAITER'S WALK

Stand straight with a dumbbell in your right hand. Raise the dumbbell over your head (like a waiter carrying a tray). Now walk forward and backward (you can mix it up). Shift the weight to your left hand halfway through the allotted time. If you can walk for longer than 1 minute, use a heavier dumbbell.

## CLOSE-HANDS PUSHUP

Assume a pushup position with your hands about 6 inches apart (your body should form a straight line from your ankles to your head). Brace your abs, squeeze your glutes, and keep your elbows tucked in against your sides as you lower yourself until your chest is about an inch from the floor. Pause, then push up to the starting position.

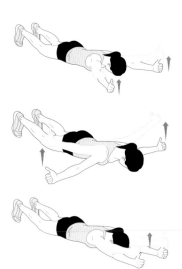

## FLOOR Y-T-I RAISES

(NOTE: Do 1 rep and start again at the beginning for the allotted time.)

Lie facedown and allow your arms to rest on the floor, each completely straight and at a 30-degree angle to your body, your palms facing each other and thumbs up (your body should resemble the letter *Y*). Raise your arms as high as you can, pause, and then lower them to the starting position.

Next move your arms so they are straight out to your sides (your body should resemble the letter *T*). Raise your arms as high as you can, pause, and then lower them to the starting position.

Now position your arms so they're straight above your shoulders (your body should resemble the letter *I*). Raise your arms as high as you can, pause, and then lower them to the starting position.

## SECOND 10

**1 MINUTE:** Rest.

**9 MINUTES:** Perform each exercise for 1 minute, cycling through the set three times.

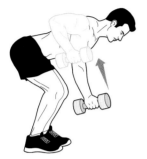

### DUMBBELL ROW

Holding a dumbbell in each hand, bend at your hips and knees and lower your torso until it's nearly parallel to the floor. Let the dumbbells hang at arm's length. Now pull the dumbbells up to the sides of your chest. Pause, then slowly lower them.

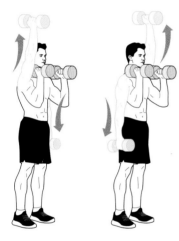

### ALTERNATING DUMBBELL CURL AND PRESS

Stand with a pair of dumbbells just outside your shoulders, arms bent, and palms facing each other. Press the right dumbbell overhead as you lower the left one to your side. Reverse the move as you return to the starting position, then press the left dumbbell overhead and lower the right. Alternate for the allotted time.

### INCHWORM

Stand tall with your legs straight. Bend over and touch the floor. Keeping your legs straight, walk your hands forward as far as you can without letting your hips sag. Then take tiny steps to walk your feet to your hands. That's 1 repetition.

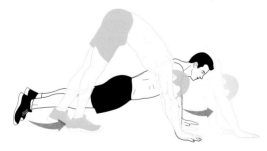

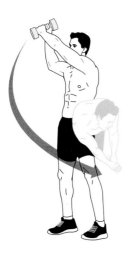

**1 MINUTE:** Rest.

**9 MINUTES:** Perform each exercise for 1 minute, cycling through the set three times.

## DUMBBELL CHOP

Hold a dumbbell with both hands above your right shoulder. Stand with your feet shoulder-width apart. Brace your core and rotate your torso to the right. While keeping your arms straight, swing the dumbbell down and to the outside of your left knee by rotating to the left and bending at your hips. Reverse the movement to return to the starting position. Halfway through the prescribed time, switch sides.

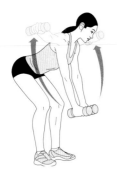

## REAR LATERAL RAISE

Grab a pair of dumbbells and bend forward at your hips until your torso is nearly parallel to the floor. Set your feet shoulder-width apart. Let the dumbbells hang straight down from your shoulders, your palms facing each other. Without moving your torso, raise your arms straight out to your sides until they're in line with your body. Pause, then slowly return to the starting position.

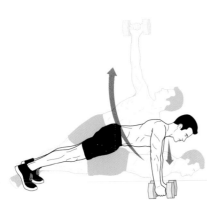

## T-PUSHUP

Grip a pair of dumbbells and assume a pushup position, using the weights as a base. Set your feet hip-width apart and your hands slightly more than shoulder-width apart. Perform a pushup. As you push yourself back up, in one fluid motion rotate the right side of your body upward as you bend your elbow and pull the right dumbbell to your torso. Then straighten your arm so the dumbbell is above your right shoulder (your body should form a *T*). Lower the dumbbell to the floor and repeat, alternating sides.

# Upper Body #3

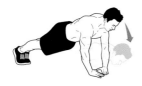

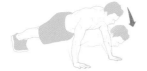

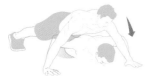

**3 MINUTES:** Do the Dynamic Warmup (page 125).

**1 MINUTE:** Rest.

**6 MINUTES:** Perform each exercise for 1 minute, cycling through the set two times.

## CHANGEUP PUSHUP

Assume a pushup position with your hands close together. Do a pushup. Next place your hands shoulder-width apart. Do a pushup. Now spread your hands twice shoulder-width apart and do a pushup. Continue reps back to the close-hands position, and repeat the cycle for the allotted time.

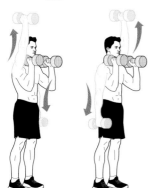

## ALTERNATING DUMBBELL CURL AND PRESS

Stand with a pair of dumbbells just outside your shoulders, arms bent, and palms facing each other. Press the right dumbbell over-head as you lower the left one to your side. Reverse the move as you return to the starting position, then press the left dumbbell overhead and lower the right. Alternate for the allotted time.

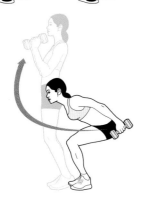

## DUMBBELL SKIER SWING

Holding a pair of dumbbells at arm's length next to your sides, stand with your knees slightly bent. Without rounding your lower back, bend at your hips as you simultaneously swing your arms backward. Now explosively thrust your hips forward and raise your torso until you're standing upright, while allowing your momentum to swing the weights up to chest level. (Don't actively lift the weights.) Swing back and forth for the allotted time.

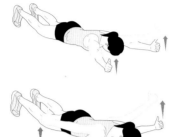

## SECOND 10

**1 MINUTE:** Rest.

**9 MINUTES:** Perform each exercise for 1 minute, cycling through the set three times.

### FLOOR Y-T-I RAISES

(NOTE: Do 1 rep and start again at the beginning for the allotted time.)

Lie facedown and allow your arms to rest on the floor, each completely straight and at a 30-degree angle to your body, your palms facing each other and thumbs up (your body should resemble the letter *Y*). Raise your arms as high as you can, pause, and then lower them to the starting position.

Next move your arms so they are straight out to your sides (your body should resemble the letter *T*). Raise your arms as high as you can, pause, and then lower them to the starting position.

Now position your arms so they're straight above your shoulders (your body should resemble the letter *I*). Raise your arms as high as you can, pause, and then lower them to the starting position.

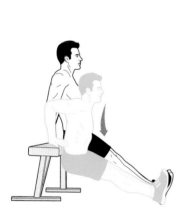

### BENCH DIP

Sit on a flat bench with your hands at your sides on the bench (or grip the sides of a chair seat). Keep your palms on the bench at all times, with your fingers facing forward and your palms down. Walk your feet out a couple of steps until your legs are extended, and lower your body just in front of the bench until your elbows are at 90 degrees. Then press through your palms to raise your body.

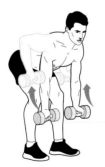

### DUMBBELL STRAIGHT-LEG DEADLIFT AND ROW

Stand with your knees slightly bent and hold a pair of dumbbells at arm's length in front of your thighs. Without rounding your lower back or changing the bend in your knees, bend at your hips and lower your torso until it's nearly parallel to the floor. Without moving your torso, pull the dumbbells up to the sides of your chest. Pause, then lower the dumbbells. Raise your torso back to the starting position.

**THIRD 10**

**1 MINUTE:** Rest.

**9 MINUTES:** Perform each exercise for 1 minute, cycling through the set three times.

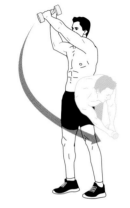

### DUMBBELL CHOP

Hold a dumbbell with both hands above your right shoulder. Stand with your feet shoulder-width apart. Brace your core and rotate your torso to the right. While keeping your arms straight, swing the dumbbell down and to the outside of your left knee by rotating to the left and bending at your hips. Reverse the movement to return to the starting position. Halfway through the prescribed time, switch sides.

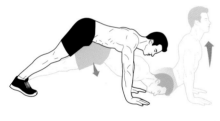

### DIVE-BOMBER PUSHUP (SOMETIMES CALLED JUDO PUSHUP)

Begin in the standard pushup position, but move your feet forward and raise your hips so your body almost forms an upside-down *V*. Keeping your hips elevated, lower your body until your chin nearly touches the floor. Lower your hips until they almost touch the floor, as you simultaneously raise your head and shoulders toward the ceiling. Reverse the movement back to the starting position and repeat.

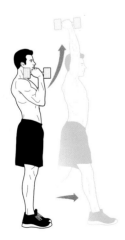

### WAITER'S WALK

Stand straight with a dumbbell in your right hand. Raise the dumbbell over your head (like a waiter carrying a tray). Now walk forward and backward (you can mix it up). Shift the weight to your left hand halfway through the allotted time. If you can walk for longer than 1 minute, use a heavier dumbbell.

# Upper Body #4

**FIRST 10**

**3 MINUTES:** Do the Dynamic Warmup (page 125).

**1 MINUTE:** Rest.

**6 MINUTES:** Perform each exercise for 1 minute, cycling through the set two times.

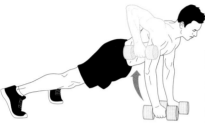

## DUMBBELL PUSHUP TO ROW

Assume a pushup position, with a dumbbell gripped in each hand as your base. Lower your body and perform 1 pushup. Now pull the right dumbbell up to the side of your chest. Pause, then lower it and repeat with the left side. That's 1 rep. Perform as many as you can in the allotted time.

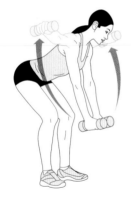

## REAR LATERAL RAISE

Grab a pair of dumbbells and bend forward at your hips until your torso is nearly parallel to the floor. Set your feet shoulder-width apart. Let the dumbbells hang straight down from your shoulders, your palms facing each other. Without moving your torso, raise your arms straight out to your sides until they're in line with your body. Pause, then slowly return to the starting position.

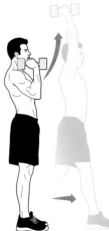

## WAITER'S WALK

Stand straight with a dumbbell in your right hand. Raise the dumbbell over your head (like a waiter carrying a tray). Now walk forward and backward (you can mix it up). Shift the weight to your left hand halfway through the allotted time. If you can walk for longer than 1 minute, use a heavier dumbbell.

## SECOND 10

**1 MINUTE:** Rest.

**9 MINUTES:** Perform each exercise for 1 minute, cycling through the set three times.

### PUSHUP-POSITION HAMMER CURL

Grip a pair of dumbbells and assume a pushup position with your palms facing each other. Brace your core and glutes. Without moving your upper arm, curl the weight in your right hand toward your right shoulder. Lower it, then repeat with your left arm. Alternate for the allotted time.

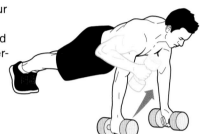

### DUMBBELL ROW

Holding a dumbbell in each hand, bend at your hips and knees and lower your torso until it's nearly parallel to the floor. Let the dumbbells hang at arm's length. Now pull the dumbbells up to the sides of your chest. Pause, then slowly lower them.

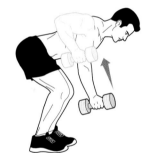

### INVERTED SHOULDER PRESS

Assume a pushup position with your feet on a bench or chair. Push your hips up so your torso is nearly perpendicular to the floor. Your hands should be slightly wider than your shoulders and your arms straight. Without changing your body posture, lower yourself until your head nearly touches the floor. Pause, then return to the starting position.

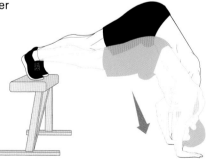

## THIRD 10

**1 MINUTE:** Rest.

**9 MINUTES:** Perform each exercise for 1 minute, cycling through the set three times.

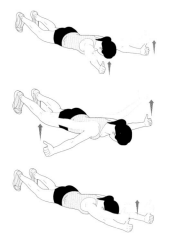

### FLOOR Y-T-I RAISES

(NOTE: Do 1 rep and start again at the beginning for the allotted time.)

Lie facedown and allow your arms to rest on the floor, each completely straight and at a 30-degree angle to your body, your palms facing each other and thumbs up (your body should resemble the letter *Y*). Raise your arms as high as you can, pause, and then lower them to the starting position.

Next move your arms so they are straight out to your sides (your body should resemble the letter *T*). Raise your arms as high as you can, pause, and then lower them to the starting position.

Now position your arms so they're straight above your shoulders (your body should resemble the letter *I*). Raise your arms as high as you can, pause, and then lower them to the starting position.

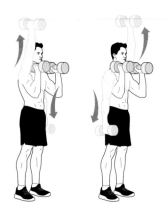

### ALTERNATING DUMBBELL CURL AND PRESS

Stand with a pair of dumbbells just outside your shoulders, arms bent, and palms facing each other. Press the right dumbbell overhead as you lower the left one to your side. Reverse the move as you return to the starting position, then press the left dumbbell overhead and lower the right. Alternate for the allotted time.

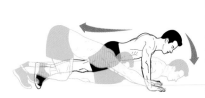

### PUSHBACK PUSHUP

Assume a pushup position with your arms straight and hands slightly wider than your shoulders. Bend at the elbows and lower your torso until your chest nearly touches the floor. Pause, then push your butt toward your ankles until your knees are bent 90 degrees. Return to the starting position and repeat.

# Upper Body #5

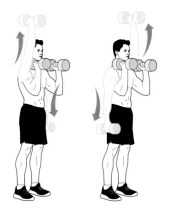

**3 MINUTES:** Do the Dynamic Warmup (page 125).

**1 MINUTE:** Rest.

**6 MINUTES:** Perform each exercise for 1 minute, cycling through the set two times.

## SINGLE-LEG PUSHUP

Assume a pushup position. While descending, lift your right leg 8 to 10 inches off the floor. Return to the starting position and descend again, this time raising your left leg. Alternate for the allotted time.

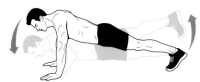
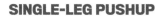

## ALTERNATING DUMBBELL CURL AND PRESS

Stand with a pair of dumbbells just outside your shoulders, arms bent, and palms facing each other. Press the right dumbbell overhead as you lower the left one to your side. Reverse the move as you return to the starting position, then press the left dumbbell overhead and lower the right. Alternate for the allotted time.

## FLOOR Y-T-I RAISES

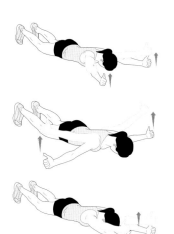

(NOTE: Do 1 rep and start again at the beginning for the allotted time.)

Lie facedown and allow your arms to rest on the floor, each completely straight and at a 30-degree angle to your body, your palms facing each other and thumbs up (your body should resemble the letter *Y*). Raise your arms as high as you can, pause, and then lower them to the starting position.

Next move your arms so they are straight out to your sides (your body should resemble the letter *T*). Raise your arms as high as you can, pause, and then lower them to the starting position.

Now position your arms so they're straight above your shoulders (your body should resemble the letter *I*). Raise your arms as high as you can, pause, and then lower them to the starting position.

## SECOND 10

**1 MINUTE:** Rest.

**9 MINUTES:** Perform each exercise for 1 minute, cycling through the set three times.

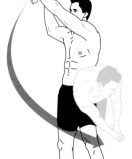

### DUMBBELL CHOP

Hold a dumbbell with both hands above your right shoulder. Stand with your feet shoulder-width apart. Brace your core and rotate your torso to the right. While keeping your arms straight, swing the dumbbell down and to the outside of your left knee by rotating to the left and bending at your hips. Reverse the movement to return to the starting position. Halfway through the prescribed time, switch sides.

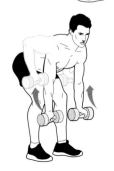

### DUMBBELL STRAIGHT-LEG DEADLIFT AND ROW

Stand with your knees slightly bent and hold a pair of dumbbells at arm's length in front of your thighs. Without rounding your lower back or changing the bend in your knees, bend at your hips and lower your torso until it's nearly parallel to the floor. Without moving your torso, pull the dumbbells up to the sides of your chest. Pause, then lower the dumbbells. Raise your torso back to the starting position.

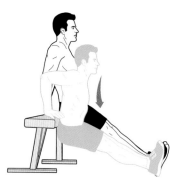

### BENCH DIP

Sit on a flat bench with your hands at your sides on the bench (or grip the sides of a chair seat). Keep your palms on the bench at all times, with your fingers facing forward and your palms down. Walk your feet out a couple of steps until your legs are extended, and lower your body just in front of the bench until your elbows are at 90 degrees. Then press through your palms to raise your body.

## THIRD 10

**1 MINUTE:** Rest.

**9 MINUTES:** Perform each exercise for 1 minute, cycling through the set three times.

### INCHWORM

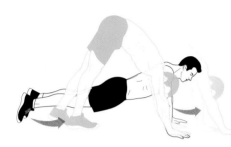

Stand tall with your legs straight. Bend over and touch the floor. Keeping your legs straight, walk your hands forward as far as you can without letting your hips sag. Then take tiny steps to walk your feet to your hands. That's 1 repetition.

### WAITER'S WALK

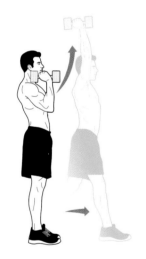

Stand straight with a dumbbell in your right hand. Raise the dumbbell over your head (like a waiter carrying a tray). Now walk forward and backward (you can mix it up). Shift the weight to your left hand halfway through the allotted time. If you can walk for longer than 1 minute, use a heavier dumbbell.

### DIVE-BOMBER PUSHUP (SOMETIMES CALLED JUDO PUSHUP)

Begin in the standard pushup position, but move your feet forward and raise your hips so your body almost forms an upside-down *V*. Keeping your hips elevated, lower your body until your chin nearly touches the floor. Lower your hips until they almost touch the floor, as you simultaneously raise your head and shoulders toward the ceiling. Reverse the movement back to the starting position and repeat.

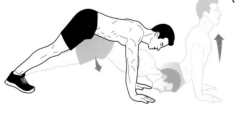

# MORE FOR THE CORE

If there's one thing I like about the term *core*, it's the nuclear connotation: that of a central power source where a reaction begins. Your core muscles (not just your "abs" but also every fiber in your torso) help generate just about any movement, especially athletic ones. A strong core is a fundamental part of a healthy kinetic chain and prevents common injuries like lower-back pain. Plus, I've noticed a phenomenon in myself and in many of the folks I treat: strong core = feeling great.

# More for the Core #1

## FIRST 10

3 **MINUTES:** Do the Dynamic Warmup (page 125).

1 **MINUTE:** Rest.

6 **MINUTES:** Perform each exercise for 1 minute, cycling through the set two times.

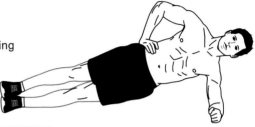

### SIDE PLANK

Lie on your left side, prop yourself up on your left forearm, and raise your hips so your body is straight from ankles to head. Hold for half the allotted time, then switch sides and repeat.

### CRAB ROLL

Sit, knees bent, with your palms and feet on the floor. Raise your hips so your body is in a straight line from your knees to your shoulders; this is the starting position. Lift your right foot and left hand and flip over to your right, placing your left hand back on the floor and kicking your right leg out behind you. (Keep it elevated.) Flip back to the starting position. That's 1 rep.

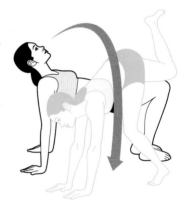

### PRONE COBRA

Lie facedown on the floor with your legs straight and your arms at your sides, palms down. Contract your glutes and lift your head, chest, arms, and legs off the floor. Simultaneously rotate your arms so your thumbs point toward the ceiling. Your hips should be the only part of your body touching the floor. Hold for a 5 count, then return to the starting position. Perform as many reps as you can in the allotted time.

**1 MINUTE:** Rest.

**9 MINUTES:** Perform each exercise for 1 minute, cycling through the set three times.

### THREE-POINT CORE TOUCH

Assume a pushup position. Quickly move your right leg forward so your right heel lands outside your right hand. Pause and return to the pushup position. Now quickly move your right leg forward so your right foot lands outside your left hand, and then return to the pushup position. That's 1 rep. Work for half the allotted time, then repeat with your left leg.

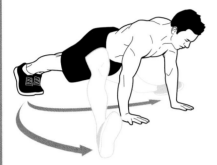

### DUMBBELL RUSSIAN TWIST

Sit on the floor, holding a dumbbell in front of your chest with both hands. Lean your torso back slightly and raise your feet off the floor. Without moving your torso, rotate the weight to your right and then to your left. Move back and forth quickly throughout the allotted time.

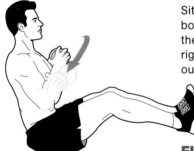

### ELEVATED BIRD DOG

Assume a pushup position and "walk" your feet forward so your knees are bent about 90 degrees and slightly above the floor. Raise your right arm and left leg until they're in line with your body. Return to the starting position, and then repeat with your left arm and right leg. Alternate arms and legs with each rep.

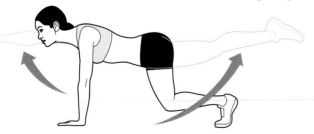

## THIRD 10

**1 MINUTE:** Rest.

**9 MINUTES:** Perform each exercise for 1 minute, cycling through the set three times.

### SINGLE-LEG, SINGLE-ARM PLANK

Assume a pushup position but with your weight on your forearms. Brace your abs, clench your glutes, and keep your body straight from head to heels. Raise your left leg and extend your right arm out in front of you. Hold for 5 seconds, then lower your arm and leg and raise your right leg/left arm for 5 seconds. Alternate for the allotted time.

### HIP-UP

Lie on your left side, your right arm extended so it's perpendicular to the floor. Prop yourself up on your left forearm and raise your hips so your body is straight from ankles to head. Lower your left hip, and then raise it again until it's in line with your body. Halfway through the allotted time, switch sides and repeat.

### LEGS-DOWN

Lie on your back, legs straight and together. Keeping your legs straight, bring them all the way up and reach for the ceiling until your butt comes off the floor. Slowly lower your legs back down almost to the floor, and then raise them back up again. Use a controlled motion throughout the exercise.

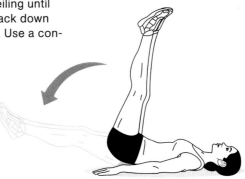

# More for the Core #2

**3 MINUTES:** Do the Dynamic Warmup (page 125).

**1 MINUTE:** Rest.

**6 MINUTES:** Perform each exercise for 1 minute, cycling through the set two times.

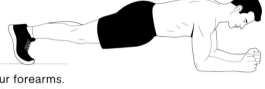

## PLANK

Assume a pushup position but with your weight on your forearms. Brace your abs, clench your glutes, and keep your body straight from head to heels.

## THE RUNNER

Lie on your back with your legs straight, elbows at your sides, and arms bent 90 degrees. This is the starting position. Lift your shoulders and back off the floor as you bring your left knee toward your chest and drive your right arm forward (as if you're running). Return to the starting position. Repeat with your right knee and left arm and alternate sides.

## HIP-UP

Lie on your left side, your right arm extended so it's perpendicular to the floor. Prop yourself up on your left forearm and raise your hips so your body is straight from ankles to head. Lower your left hip, and then raise it again until it's in line with your body. Halfway through the allotted time, switch sides and repeat.

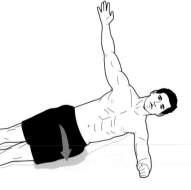

## SECOND 10

**1 MINUTE:** Rest.

**9 MINUTES:** Perform each exercise for 1 minute, cycling through the set three times.

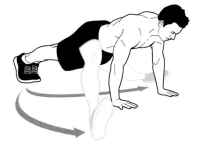

### THREE-POINT CORE TOUCH

Assume a pushup position. Quickly move your right leg forward so your right heel lands outside your right hand. Pause and return to the pushup position. Now quickly move your right leg forward so your right foot lands outside your left hand, and then return to the pushup position. That's 1 rep. Work for half the allotted time, then repeat with your left leg.

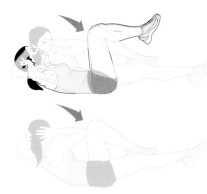

### BICYCLE CRUNCH

Lie faceup with your hips and knees bent 90 degrees so that your lower legs are parallel to the floor. Clasp your hands behind your head. Lift your shoulders off the floor and hold them there. Twist your upper body to the right as you pull your right knee in as fast as you can until it touches your left elbow. Simultaneously straighten your left leg. Return to the starting position and repeat to the other side.

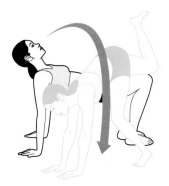

### CRAB ROLL

Sit, knees bent, with your palms and feet on the floor. Raise your hips so your body is in a straight line from your knees to your shoulders; this is the starting position. Lift your right foot and left hand and flip over to your right, placing your left hand back on the floor and kicking your right leg out behind you. (Keep it elevated.) Flip back to the starting position. That's 1 rep.

## THIRD 10

**1 MINUTE:** Rest.

**9 MINUTES:** Perform each exercise for 1 minute, cycling through the set three times.

## SIDE PLANK

Lie on your left side, prop yourself up on your left forearm, and raise your hips so your body is straight from ankles to head. Hold for half the allotted time, then switch sides and repeat.

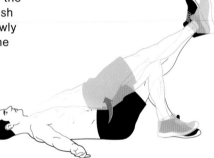

## SINGLE-LEG HIP RAISE

Lie on your back with your left knee bent and left foot flat on the floor. Raise your right leg so it's in line with your left thigh. Push your hips up, keeping your right leg elevated. Pause, then slowly return to the starting position. Switch legs halfway through the allotted time.

## FIGURE 8

Lie on your back with your arms at your sides, palms down. Raise your legs so they form a 45-degree angle with the floor. Now make big, looping circles with your legs, first to your left and then to your right, forming a sideways figure 8. That's 1 rep.

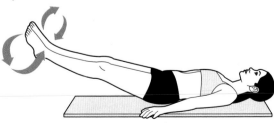

# More for the Core #3

**3 MINUTES:** Do the Dynamic Warmup (page 125).

**1 MINUTE:** Rest.

**6 MINUTES:** Perform each exercise for 1 minute, cycling through the set two times.

## HIP RAISE

Lie faceup on the floor with your knees bent and your feet flat on the floor. Raise your hips so your body forms a straight line from your shoulders to your knees. Clench your glutes as you reach the top of the movement. Pause, then lower your body back to the starting position.

## ELEVATED BIRD DOG

Assume a pushup position and "walk" your feet forward so your knees are bent about 90 degrees and slightly above the floor. Raise your right arm and left leg until they're in line with your body. Return to the starting position, and then repeat with your left arm and right leg. Alternate arms and legs with each rep.

## PRONE COBRA

Lie facedown on the floor with your legs straight and your arms at your sides, palms down. Contract your glutes and lift your head, chest, arms, and legs off the floor. Simultaneously rotate your arms so your thumbs point toward the ceiling. Your hips should be the only part of your body touching the floor. Hold for a 5 count, then return to the starting position. Perform as many reps as you can in the allotted time.

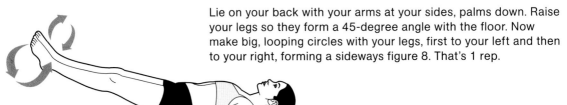

## SECOND 10

**1 MINUTE:** Rest.

**9 MINUTES:** Perform each exercise for 1 minute, cycling through the set three times.

### FIGURE 8

Lie on your back with your arms at your sides, palms down. Raise your legs so they form a 45-degree angle with the floor. Now make big, looping circles with your legs, first to your left and then to your right, forming a sideways figure 8. That's 1 rep.

### PLANK

Assume a pushup position but with your weight on your forearms. Brace your abs, clench your glutes, and keep your body straight from head to heels.

### THE RUNNER

Lie on your back with your legs straight, elbows at your sides, and arms bent 90 degrees. This is the starting position. Lift your shoulders and back off the floor as you bring your left knee toward your chest and drive your right arm forward (as if you're running). Return to the starting position. Repeat with your right knee and left arm and alternate sides.

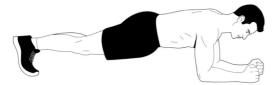

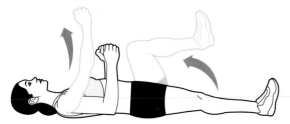

## THIRD 10

**1 MINUTE:** Rest.

**9 MINUTES:** Perform each exercise for 1 minute, cycling through the set three times.

### SINGLE-LEG SIDE PLANK

Lie on your side and use your forearm to support your body. Raise your hips until your body forms a straight line from shoulders to ankles. Then raise your top leg as high as you can, holding it there for the duration of the exercise. Halfway through the prescribed time, switch sides.

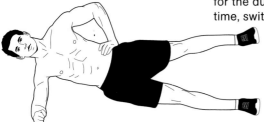

### DUMBBELL RUSSIAN TWIST

Sit on the floor, holding a dumbbell in front of your chest with both hands. Lean your torso back slightly and raise your feet off the floor. Without moving your torso, rotate the weight to your right and then to your left. Move back and forth quickly throughout the allotted time.

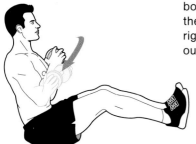

### LEGS-DOWN

Lie on your back, legs straight and together. Keeping your legs straight, bring them all the way up and reach for the ceiling until your butt comes off the floor. Slowly lower your legs back down almost to the floor, and then raise them back up again. Use a controlled motion throughout the exercise.

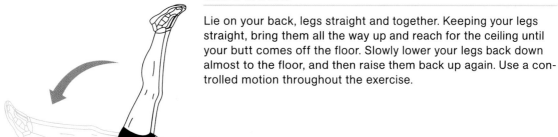

# More for the Core #4

**3 MINUTES:** Do the Dynamic Warmup (page 125).

**1 MINUTE:** Rest.

**6 MINUTES:** Perform each exercise for 1 minute, cycling through the set two times.

## SINGLE-LEG, SINGLE-ARM PLANK

Assume a pushup position but with your weight on your forearms. Brace your abs, clench your glutes, and keep your body straight from head to heels. Raise your left leg and extend your right arm out in front of you. Hold for 5 seconds, then lower your arm and leg and raise your right leg/left arm for 5 seconds. Alternate for the allotted time.

## BICYCLE CRUNCH

Lie faceup with your hips and knees bent 90 degrees so that your lower legs are parallel to the floor. Clasp your hands behind your head. Lift your shoulders off the floor and hold them there. Twist your upper body to the right as you pull your right knee in as fast as you can until it touches your left elbow. Simultaneously straighten your left leg. Return to the starting position and repeat to the other side.

## PRONE COBRA

Lie facedown on the floor with your legs straight and your arms at your sides, palms down. Contract your glutes and lift your head, chest, arms, and legs off the floor. Simultaneously rotate your arms so your thumbs point toward the ceiling. Your hips should be the only part of your body touching the floor. Hold for a 5 count, then return to the starting position. Perform as many reps as you can in the allotted time.

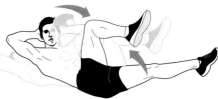

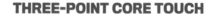

## SECOND 10

**1 MINUTE:** Rest.

**9 MINUTES:** Perform each exercise for 1 minute, cycling through the set three times.

### THREE-POINT CORE TOUCH

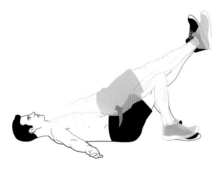

Assume a pushup position. Quickly move your right leg forward so your right heel lands outside your right hand. Pause and return to the pushup position. Now quickly move your right leg forward so your right foot lands outside your left hand, and then return to the pushup position. That's 1 rep. Work for half the allotted time, then repeat with your left leg.

### SINGLE-LEG HIP RAISE

Lie on your back with your left knee bent and your left foot flat on the floor. Raise your right leg so it's in line with your left thigh. Push your hips up, keeping your right leg elevated. Pause, then slowly return to the starting position. Switch legs halfway through the allotted time.

### CRAB ROLL

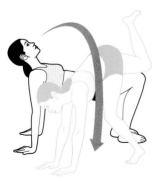

Sit, knees bent, with your palms and feet on the floor. Raise your hips so your body is in a straight line from your knees to your shoulders; this is the starting position. Lift your right foot and left hand and flip over to your right, placing your left hand back on the floor and kicking your right leg out behind you. (Keep it elevated.) Flip back to the starting position. That's 1 rep.

## THIRD 10

**1 MINUTE:** Rest.

**9 MINUTES:** Perform each exercise for 1 minute, cycling through the set three times.

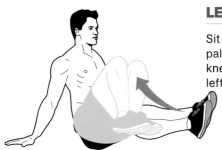

### LEG TUCK AND TWIST

Sit on the floor, leaning back 45 degrees, your legs straight and palms on the floor behind you. Lift your legs off the floor. Pull your knees toward your left shoulder as you twist your torso to your left. Return to the starting position and repeat to your right.

### SINGLE-LEG SIDE PLANK

Lie on your side and use your forearm to support your body. Raise your hips until your body forms a straight line from shoulders to ankles. Then raise your top leg as high as you can, holding it there for the duration of the exercise. Halfway through the prescribed time, switch sides.

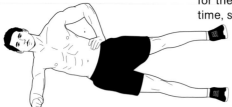

### FIGURE 8

Lie on your back with your arms at your sides, palms down. Raise your legs so they form a 45-degree angle with the floor. Now make big, looping circles with your legs, first to your left and then to your right, forming a sideways figure 8. That's 1 rep.

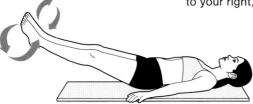

# More for the Core #5

## FIRST 10

**3 MINUTES:** Do the Dynamic Warmup (page 125).

**1 MINUTE:** Rest.

**6 MINUTES:** Perform each exercise for 1 minute, cycling through the set two times.

## PLANK

Assume a pushup position but with your weight on your forearms. Brace your abs, clench your glutes, and keep your body straight from head to heels.

## HIP-UP

Lie on your left side, your right arm extended so it's perpendicular to the floor. Prop yourself up on your left forearm and raise your hips so your body is straight from ankles to head. Lower your left hip, and then raise it again until it's in line with your body. Halfway through the allotted time, switch sides and repeat.

## FIGURE 8

Lie on your back with your arms at your sides, palms down. Raise your legs so they form a 45-degree angle with the floor. Now make big, looping circles with your legs, first to your left and then to your right, forming a sideways figure 8. That's 1 rep.

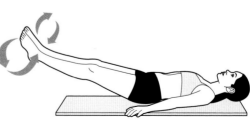

## SECOND 10

**1 MINUTE:** Rest.

**9 MINUTES:** Perform each exercise for 1 minute, cycling through the set three times.

### ELEVATED BIRD DOG

Assume a pushup position and "walk" your feet forward so your knees are bent about 90 degrees and slightly above the floor. Raise your right arm and left leg until they're in line with your body. Return to the starting position, and then repeat with your left arm and right leg. Alternate arms and legs with each rep.

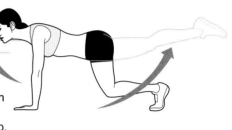

### BICYCLE CRUNCH

Lie faceup with your hips and knees bent 90 degrees so that your lower legs are parallel to the floor. Clasp your hands behind your head. Lift your shoulders off the floor and hold them there. Twist your upper body to the right as you pull your right knee in as fast as you can until it touches your left elbow. Simultaneously straighten your left leg. Return to the starting position and repeat to the other side.

### PRONE COBRA

Lie facedown on the floor with your legs straight and your arms at your sides, palms down. Contract your glutes and lift your head, chest, arms, and legs off the floor. Simultaneously rotate your arms so your thumbs point toward the ceiling. Your hips should be the only part of your body touching the floor. Hold for a 5 count, then return to the starting position. Perform as many reps as you can in the allotted time.

**THIRD 10**

**1 MINUTE:** Rest.

**9 MINUTES:** Perform each exercise for 1 minute, cycling through the set three times.

### SIDE PLANK

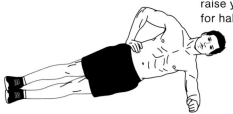

Lie on your left side, prop yourself up on your left forearm, and raise your hips so your body is straight from ankles to head. Hold for half the allotted time, then switch sides and repeat.

### THE RUNNER

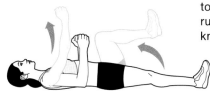

Lie on your back with your legs straight, elbows at your sides, and arms bent 90 degrees. This is the starting position. Lift your shoulders and back off the floor as you bring your left knee toward your chest and drive your right arm forward (as if you're running). Return to the starting position. Repeat with your right knee and left arm and alternate sides.

### DUMBBELL RUSSIAN TWIST

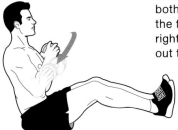

Sit on the floor, holding a dumbbell in front of your chest with both hands. Lean your torso back slightly and raise your feet off the floor. Without moving your torso, rotate the weight to your right and then to your left. Move back and forth quickly through-out the allotted time.

# ENDNOTES

## CHAPTER 1

1 Burleson, M. A., H. S. O'Bryant, M. H. Stone, M. A. Collins et al., "Effect of Weight Training Exercise and Treadmill Exercise on Postexercise Oxygen Consumption," *Medicine and Science in Sports and Exercise* 30, no. 4 (1998): 518–22.

2 Osterberg, K. L., and C. L. Melby, "Effect of Acute Resistance Exercise on Postexercise Oxygen Consumption and Resting Metabolic Rate in Young Women," *International Journal of Sport Nutrition and Exercise Metabolism* 10 (September 2000): 360.

3 Matsuo, T., K. Ohkawra, S. Seino, S. Nobutake et al., "Cardiorespiratory Fitness Level Correlates Inversely with Excess Post-Exercise Oxygen Consumption after Aerobic-Type Interval Training," *BMC Research Notes* 5 (2012): 646. Published online 2012 Nov 21. doi:10.1186/1756-0500-5-646.

4 Gillen, J. B., M. E. Percival, L. E. Skelly, B. J. Martin et al, "Three Minutes of All-Out Intermittent Exercise per Week Increases Skeletal Muscle Oxidative Capacity and Improves Cardiometabolic Health," *PLOS ONE* 9, no. 11 (2014): e111489. doi:10.1371/journal.pone.0111489.

5 Gillen, J. B., B. J. Martin, M. J. MacInnis, L. E. Skelly et al., "Twelve Weeks of Sprint Interval Training Improves Indices of Cardiometabolic Health Similar to Traditional Endurance Training Despite a Five-Fold Lower Exercise Volume and Time Commitment," *PLOS ONE* 11, no. 4 (2016): e0154075. doi:10.1371/journal.pone.0154075.

6 Moller Madsen, S., A. C. Thorup, K. Overgaard, and P. Bendix Jeppesen, "High Intensity Interval Training Improves Glycaemic Control and Pancreatic β Cell Function of Type 2 Diabetes Patients," *PLOS ONE* 10, no. 8 (2015): e0133286. Published online 2015 Aug 10. doi:10.1371/journal.pone.0133286. PMCID: PMC4530878.

7 Adams, O. P., "The Impact of Brief High-Intensity Exercise on Blood Glucose Levels," *Diabetes, Metabolic Syndrome and Obesity: Targets and Therapy* 6 (2013): 113–22. Published online 2013 Feb 27. doi: 10.2147/DMSO. S29222. PMCID: PMC3587394.

8 Ahmadizad, S. A., S. Avansar, K. Ebrahim, M. Avandi et al., "The Effects of Short-Term High-Intensity Interval Training vs. Moderate-Intensity Continuous Training on Plasma Levels of Nesfatin-1 and Inflammatory Markers," *Hormone Molecular Biology and Clinical Investigation* 21, no. 3 (March 2015): 165–73. doi: 10.1515/hmbci-2014-0038.

9 Buckley, S., K. Knapp, A. Lackie, C. Lewry et al., "Multimodal High-intensity Interval Training Increases Muscle Function and Metabolic Performance in Females," *Applied Physiology, Nutrition, and Metabolism* 40, no. 11 (November 2015): 1157–62. doi: 10.1139/apnm-2015-0238. Epub 2015 Jul 28.

10 Jung, M.E. J. E. Bourne, and J. P. Little, "Where Does HIT Fit? An Examination of the Affective Response to High-Intensity Intervals in Comparison to Continuous Moderate- and Continuous Vigorous-Intensity Exercise in the Exercise Intensity-Affect Continuum," *PLOS ONE* 9, no. 12 (2014): e114541. doi:10.1371/journal.pone.0114541.

11 Kilpatrick, M. W., N. Martinez, J. P. Little, M. E. Jung et al., "Impact of High-Intensity Interval Duration on Perceived Exertion," *Medicine and Science in Sports and Exercise* 47, no. 5 (May 2015): 1038–45. doi: 10.1249/MSS.0000000000000495.

12 Gliemann, L., T. P. Gunnarsson, Y. Hellsten, and J. Bangsbo, "10-20-30 Training Increases Performance and Lowers Blood Pressure and VEGF in Runners," *Scandinavian Journal of Medicine and Science in Sports* 25, no. 5 (2015): e479-89. doi: 10.1111/sms.12356. Epub 2014 Dec 1.

13  Mikkola, J., V. Vesterinen, R. Taipale, B. Capostagno et al., "Effect of Resistance Training Regimens on Treadmill Running and Neuromuscular Performance in Recreational Endurance Runners," KIHU-Research Institute for Olympic Sports, Jyväskylä, Finland. *Journal of Sports Sciences* 29, no. 13 (October 2011): 1359–71. Epub 2011 Aug 22.

14  Aagaard, P., J. L. Andersen, M. Bennekou, B. Larsson et al., "Effects of Resistance Training on Endurance Capacity and Muscle Fiber Composition in Young Top-level Cyclists," *Scandinavian Journal of Medicine and Science in Sports* 21, no. 6 (December 2011): e298-307. doi: 10.1111/j.1600-0838.2010.01283.x. Epub 2011 Mar 1.

## CHAPTER 2

1   Sui, X., L. Hongjuan, J. Li, L. Zhang, L. Chen et al., "Percentage of Deaths Attributable to Poor Cardiovascular Health Lifestyle Factors: Findings from the Aerobics Center Longitudinal Study," *Epidemiology Research International* 2013 (2103): Article ID 437465, 9 pages. doi:10.1155/2013/437465.

2   D'Mello, M. J., S. A. Ross, M. Briel, S. S. Anand et al., "Association between Shortened Leukocyte Telomere Length and Cardiometabolic Outcomes: Systematic Review and Meta-Analysis," *Circulation: Cardiovascular Genetics* 8, no. 1 (February 2015): 82–90. Published online before print: November 18 2014, doi: 10.1161/CIRCGENETICS.113.000485.

3   Cherkas, L. F., J. L. Hunkin, B. S. Kato et al., "The Association between Physical Activity in Leisure Time and Leukocyte Telomere Length," *Archives of Internal Medicine* 168, no. 2 (2008): 154–58. doi:10.1001/archinternmed.2007.39.

4   Loprinzi, P. D., J. P. Loenneke, and E. H. Blackburn, "Movement-Based Behaviors and Leukocyte Telomere Length among US Adults," *Medicine and Science in Sports and Exercise* 47, no. 11 (2015): 2347–52. doi: 10.1249/MSS.0000000000000695.

5   Silva, L. C., A L. de Araújo, J. R. Fernandes, Mde. S. Matias et al., "Moderate and Intense Exercise Lifestyles Attenuate the Effects of Aging on Telomere Length and the Survival and Composition of T Cell Subpopulations," *Age (Dordr)* 38, no. 1 (February 2016): 24.

6   Ibid.

7   Saßenroth, D., A. Meyer, B. Salewsky, M. Kroh et al., "Sports and Exercise at Different Ages and Leukocyte Telomere Length in Later Life—Data from the Berlin Aging Study II (BASE-II)." *PLOS ONE* 10, no. 12 (December 2, 2015).

8   Mosallanezhad, Z., N. Hojatollah, A. Nikbakht, and A. Gaeini, "The Effect of High-Intensity Interval Training on Telomerase Activity of Leukocytes in Sedentary Young Women," *International Journal of Analytical, Pharmaceutical, and Biomedical Sciences* 3, no. 5 (November 2014). Copyrights ©2014 ISSN:2278-0246. Coden: IJAPBS www .ijapbs.com.

9   Fotuhi, M., D. Do, and C. Jack, "Modifiable Factors That Alter the Size of the Hippocampus with Ageing," *Nature Reviews Neurology* 8, no. 4 (2012): 189–202. 10.1038/nrneurol.2012.27.

10  Van Praag, H., "Exercise and the Brain: Something to Chew On," *Trends in Neuroscience* 32, no. 5 (2009): 283–90. doi:10.1016/j.tins.2008.12.007.

11  Weinberg, L., A. Hasni, M. Shinohara, A. Duartea, "A Single Bout of Resistance Exercise Can Enhance Episodic Memory Performance," *Acta Psychologica* 153 (November 2014): 13–19.

12  Burzynska, A. Z., L. Chaddock-Heyman, M. W. Voss, C. N. Wong et al, "Physical Activity and Cardiorespiratory Fitness Are Beneficial for White Matter in Low-Fit Older Adults," *PLOS ONE* 9, no. 9 (2014): e107413. doi:10.1371/journal.pone.0107413.

13  Erickson, K. I., M. W. Voss, R. S. Prakash et al., "Exercise Training Increases Size of Hippocampus and Improves Memory," *Proceedings of the National Academy of Sciences of the United States of America* 108, no. 7 (2011): 3017–22. doi:10.1073/pnas.1015950108.

14  Chételat, G., V. L. Villemagne, K. E. Pike, J.-C. Baron et al., "Larger Temporal Volume in Elderly with High versus Low Beta-Amyloid Deposition," *Brain: A Journal of Neurology* 133, no. 11 (August 2010): 3349–58. doi: http://dx.doi.org/10.1093/brain/awq187 3349-3358. First published online: 25 August 2010.

## CHAPTER 5

1  Barbosa Barreto de Brito, L., D. Rabelo Ricardo, D. Sardinha Mendes Soares de Araújo, P. Santos Ramos et al., "Ability to Sit and Rise from the Floor as a Predictor of All-Cause Mortality," *European Journal of Preventive Cardiology* 21, no. 7 (July 2014): 892–98.

# ACKNOWLEDGMENTS

I'd like to thank all of the many people who have helped my simultaneous career paths of physician, fitness instructor, and author as I strive to make a positive mark in the world.

On the book side of my life, my Rodale family, including editor extraordinaire Mark Weinstein, the Rodale book group, and the company at large, across all brands and platforms, has been immensely helpful. I'm so lucky to have fallen into such a perfect match, a group of people who not only educate the world about the benefits of health and wellness but also teach me with every interaction. I'm so deeply honored and inspired to be part of the Rodale family and greatly appreciate their help and support as I try to disseminate my knowledge. I could never have imagined a better place to publish my books and information.

I'm deeply indebted to Mike Zimmerman, whose organizational and editorial skills are invaluable. It is such a pleasure to work with him on a second book. Zim, you are amazing.

On the doctor side of my life, the Hospital for Special Surgery, where I've worked my entire career as a sports medicine physician, continues to lead the world in all aspects of sports medicine and orthopedics. It was my greatest professional triumph to end up in such a uniquely supportive and forward-thinking hospital to build my medical career. I owe my colleagues and friends at HSS every bit of my success. They are each the top in their respective fields and they make me a better physician every day through their brilliance. The daily workings of my medical practice could never be possible without the tireless efforts of my office staff and nurses, who help keep my medical practice running smoothly. I can never thank you enough for your help.

On the athlete and fitness instructor side of my life, I'm so appreciative to the many companies, including BBDO, Equinox, Johnson and Johnson, TYR sports, Timex Sports, Inov8, Asics, Headsweats, Chloe's Fruit, VitaCoco, the Intrepid Museum, Central Park Conservancy, Canyon Ranch, Rancho La Puerta, Lifetime Fitness, Pure Yoga, Mile High Run Club, ESPN-W, JBL Audio, and many others who have helped me combine the worlds of fitness and medicine. Each of you has contributed to our efforts to build and grow the IronStrength brand, the megaphone through which we try and convince the world that health-care professionals should not only treat disease but should also prevent it using the medicine of exercise.

This list is just a small fraction of the many people who have taken their time and effort to make me better in all aspects of my life. I am deeply appreciative of you all, thank you.

# INDEX

Boldface page references indicate illustrations. <u>Underscored</u> references indicate boxed text.

Jordan D. Metzl, MD, is an award-winning sports medicine physician at the industry-leading Hospital for Special Surgery in New York City. With a medical practice of more than 20,000 patients, Dr. Metzl treats athletic patients of all ages in his New York and Connecticut offices, the focus being safe and healthy participation to activity. When he's not treating knees, backs, shoulders, or other injured body parts, Dr. Metzl is moving. He's authored five books including *The Athlete's Book of Home Remedies, The Exercise Cure, and Dr. Jordan Metzl's Running Strong.* He created the IronStrength workout, which has been performed by more than 10 million athletes around the world, and also founded the IronStrength community fitness program, which runs free, community-based fitness programs to promote health and wellness. In addition to his medical practice, books, and fitness classes, Dr. Metzl is a 14-time Ironman and 33-time marathon finisher (and still going). He lives, works, and works out in New York City.

**Mike Zimmerman** is the author or coauthor of more than 30 books, including *The Athlete's Book of Home Remedies* with Jordan D. Metzl, MD. He is a former senior and contributing editor of *Men's Health* magazine.